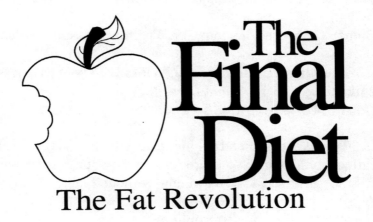

The Final Diet

The Fat Revolution

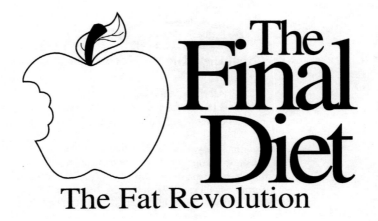

The Final Diet
The Fat Revolution

by
Michael Chatterson M.D., C.C.F.P.
Linda Chatterson Reg.N.

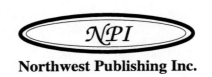

NPI

Northwest Publishing Inc.

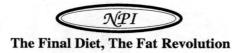

The Final Diet, The Fat Revolution

PRINTING HISTORY
First Printing 1994

ISBN: 1-56901-172-9

NPI books are published by Northwest Publishing Incorporated,
5949 South 350 West, Salt Lake City, Utah 84107.
The name "NPI" and the "NPI" logo are trademarks belonging to
Northwest Publishing Incorporated.

PRINTED IN THE UNITED STATES OF AMERICA.
10 9 8 7 6 5 4 3 2 1

You should discuss your specific dietary and fitness needs with your doctor before starting the final diet and exercise program. If you suffer from serious medical problems, modifications to the program may be necessary.

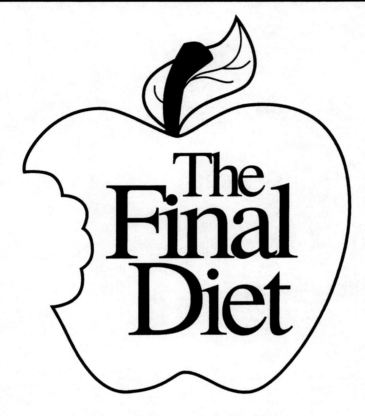

The Final Diet

The Fat Revolution

CONTENTS

PREFACE   IX

ACKNOWLEDGMENTS   XI

INTRODUCTION   XIII

A TIME FOR ACTION   1

THE INSIDE STORY—HOW THE BODY USES FOOD   3

TWO INGREDIENTS FOR SUCCESS   19

THE FINAL DIET 'GAME PLAN'   21

GREAT FOODS—PART 1:   32
       THE COMPLEX CARBOHYDRATES—THE STUFF OF LIFE

GREAT FOODS—PART 2:   41
       TURKEY, CHICKEN (AND FISH)—BIRDS OF PARADISE

GREAT FOODS—PART 3:   46
       LOW FAT DAIRY PRODUCTS—HEALTHY PROTEIN

THE FAT TRAPS—HOW TO BEAT THEM   50

A REVIEW—SMART SUBSTITUTIONS   61

SURVIVAL KIT FOR DINING OUT   63

EXERCISE—THE SECOND ESSENTIAL   65

CHOLESTEROL—A FEW WORDS OF ADVICE   72

THE FINAL DIET—LET'S GO!!   74

COMMON QUESTIONS   75

MEAL PLANS—TWO WEEKS OF GREAT DINING!   78

THE FINAL DIET—RECIPES   91

FOOD LISTS—INDEX   161

WRAP-UP   169

BIBLIOGRAPHY   171

INDEX   175

PREFACE

A beacon of hope shines for the millions who struggle daily with being overweight. This book was written to share the knowledge and the weight loss method that sustain that hope. Permanent weight loss and fitness are possible for all of us, without hunger.

Linda and I discovered the benefits of low-fat living several years ago. I was gamely fighting the expanding girth of impending mid-life. Our journey from the science, to the food, to the grocery store, to the kitchen, to the table and to the gym has been a revelation. We take that journey in this book. At the end of that journey we discover normal weight and fitness.

Researching and writing the final diet has been an adventure. We have discovered that most people don't understand what food really is, and suffer the consequences. Weight loss has become confused with starvation.

This book unlocks the secrets of food. Armed with clear knowledge about food, particularly fat, we combat the spectre of obesity. We discover that we can eat well while restoring our bodies to health.

If you are overweight, or if you simply yearn for a more vibrant way of life—there is hope! This book was written to restore your hope in achieving normal weight and fitness and to lead you, step by step, to that goal.

ACKNOWLEDGMENTS

Our heartfelt thanks to Cathy Prowd, "computer wizard", for her excellent work and enthusiasm despite countless revisions of this manuscript.

Special thanks are given to our friends, Brian and Helen Barrie, George Dunne, Deirdre Ellis, Marion Legge, Dr. Shane Peng and Dr. Roger Skinner for their valuable suggestions and feedback in this enjoyable project. The valuable support and suggestions of dietitians Ellen van der Meer and Carol Hudgins are greatly appreciated. Thank you to Peter Reid of Austin Graphics for his artistic guidance.

We greatly appreciate the time and interest in the book by our 40 (or so) sample readers—lay people, nurses, dietitians, family physicians, cardiologists and lipid specialists. Your comments, and endorsements, are critical to the success of the book.

We thank the talented people at Northwest Publications Inc. for their enthusiasm and hard work.

And lastly, thank you to our kids for trying all that "new food", and for the brilliant cover design.

WEIGHTS AND MEASURES	
WEIGHTS	1 gm = 1/30 oz 1000 gm = 1 kilogram 1 lb = 16 oz = .45 kilogram
MEASURES	3 tsp (t) = 1 tbsp (T) = 15 ml 2 T = 1 oz = 30 ml 16 T = 8 oz = 1 cup = 240 ml = 1/4 litre 2 cups = 1 pint 2 pints = 1 quart
MEASURES/WEIGHTS	1 cup (8 oz / 240 ml) of water weighs 240 grams 1 oz (30 ml) of water weighs 30 grams

I don't care about the cheese,
I just want out of the trap!
—old Spanish proverb

Introduction

A Fat Crisis

30% of adult North Americans, and almost as many Europeans are obese. Obesity is defined as having a body weight more than 20% over ideal.

Scientists have now proven three sobering facts:

Fact: High-fat diets are the *main* cause of obesity.

Fact: Obesity and high-fat diets result in suffering and death from a myriad of diseases including heart disease, cancer, strokes, high blood pressure and diabetes.

Fact: A low-fat diet will restore normal body weight and reduce suffering and death from the diseases associated with the North American high fat diet.

The citizens of the world's richest nations are poisoning themselves with *fat*. The needless suffering and health care costs associated with that abuse has created a *fat crisis*.

Relief at Last!

Rescue from the fat crisis has appeared from two directions—from the *science of nutrition* and from the *food industry*.

Nutritional scientists know exactly what nourishment our bodies need to thrive. We know what proportions of foodstuffs—fat, protein and carbohydrate—are necessary for a lean, efficient human machine. Carbohydrates—rice, potatoes, bread, pasta, beans, vegetables and fruit—are the ideal foods that fuel our engines. A human body fed 60% of its calories as carbohydrates will be lean and mean. Fat, in excess, results in obesity and disease. The precise knowledge of the body's nutritional needs is a vital weapon in attacking the fat problem.

The *food industry*, armed with knowledge is reacting to the fat crisis. Supermarket shelves feature new and delicious low fat alternatives to common high fat foods. Low fat foods retain the taste and the texture of their high fat cousins without excessive calories and fat content. An excellent example is no-fat mayonnaise which has the same look and taste as regular mayonnaise with 1/8 the calories (12 versus 99 per tablespoon) and no fat.

In the next five years the food industry will produce hundreds of low fat foods that will help us apply our knowledge of nutrition. Armed with modern scientific nutritional knowledge and wonderful low fat foods, *we can eat well and be slim!*

THE FINAL DIET

Most people hate the word *diet*. The word likely was derived from two words, *die* and *trying*! You won't die trying the Final Diet. You will thrive from the combination of great food and exercise. And, most importantly, you won't be hungry!

95% of all diets fail. Diet failure means being at the same weight or higher after one year. None of us would buy a car with a 95% chance of engine failure in a year. The Final Diet breaks the pattern of failure that many of us have experienced. The Final Diet stimulates a permanent behavior change in how we use food in our lives. It combines healthy, scientific weight loss with an exercise program written for real people, not Olympians.

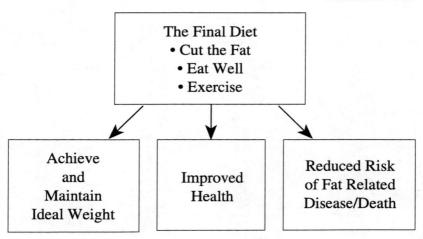

TAKE COURAGE

We get older. Our weight climbs. Our fitness slips away. It is easy to become despondent, to give up. Don't give up! Take courage! This book contains the knowledge and the road map to a lean, fit body. Join us on the journey.

Chapter 1

A Time for Action

The scale said 254 pounds!

As a 45 year old family doctor, who had spent 20 years helping *other* people with health problems, I was shocked. What was I doing to my body?

At six feet, two inches, I was the smallest male in a family of big people. I exercised daily—squash, fitness, cycling! Cottage cheese lunches and light breakfasts were the norm. Never more than one piece of pie. I was big boned, muscular—but 254 pounds!

To make matters worse, two other problems soon unmasked their hideous faces. My blood pressure was 145/96—high enough to require treatment. Secondly, my cholesterol level was elevated. Soon I would be clutching my chest with agonizing chest pain. I'd seen the landscape unfold a hundred times. With the three risk factors that I had collected—obesity, high blood pressure, and high cholesterol—the probability of heart disease was staggering.

Action!

Linda and I began an extensive study of the current knowledge of diet, nutrition, exercise and human metabolism (how the body uses food). We studied the modern theories about the causes of obesity and high blood pressure and elevated cholesterol. We learned about food. We spent hours in supermarkets, exploring the shelves, reading labels and comparing products. We experimented with food and created or modified hundreds of recipes. We tried them ourselves and shared them with friends. We discovered the benefits of a low fat, high carbohydrate diet combined with a regular, rational exercise program. My weight dropped...10, 20, 30, 40, 45 pounds! My blood pressure returned to normal (120/78). My cholesterol dropped below normal!

I'm now lean and fit again! I maintained all of the benefits of my new life style for over a year.

This book was written to share *The Final Diet* with you:

- Understand food and how the body uses it.
- Identify a reasonable weight goal.
- Learn how to feed your body to reach your goal.
- Prepare satisfying and delicious low fat meals.
- Learn to exercise in a healthy fashion to achieve fitness and your ideal weight.

Chapter 2

The Inside Story—How the Body Uses Food

All *food* is made up of a mixture of three food types—*fat, protein and carbohydrate*. The energy the body captures from food is measured in calories. The average 150 lb. person needs 2500 calories per day. Food quantities are usually measured in volumes (8 oz. of water make 1 cup) or weights (1 liquid ounce of water weighs 30 grams).

Vital facts in our quest for health:

> - 1 gram of fat has 9 calories of food energy
> - 1 gram of protein has 4 calories of food energy
> - 1 gram of carbohydrate has 4 calories of food energy

Fatty foods are stuffed with calories! One gram of fat has over twice the calories of one gram of protein or carbohydrate. Call this *the 9 to 4 rule*.

Foods have a mixture of fat, protein and carbohydrate

Most foods have a mixture of three food types. The table below illustrates how some foods, like the humble apple, are entirely carbohydrate. Other foods, such as an egg mcmuffin contain calories from fat, protein and carbohydrate.

3

FOOD	FAT CALORIES	PROTEIN CALORIES	CARBOHYDRATE CALORIES	TOTAL CALORIES
medium apple			80	80
egg mcmuffin	140	80	120	340
1 slice raisin bread	9	9	52	52
2 oz. cheddar cheese	170	56	4	230

Foods with low fat content (the 9 to 4 rule) will have lower calories per gram. The body needs all three types of food—fat, protein, and carbohydrate.

FAT: THE FACTS ABOUT FAT

Seconds after we finish the last french fry, our gut starts digesting the fat content of our meal. Special digestive proteins called enzymes split fat molecules into smaller components that pass through the gut wall into the blood stream. After a high fat meal, the blood is loaded with fat molecules. The body has two choices. It can burn the fat as fuel or it can store it in fat cells for future use, like a bear about to hibernate. Since the body finds fat a difficult fuel to break down, it stores most of the fat. Only during prolonged exercise will the body turn to fat cells for stored fat to burn for energy. The diagram below illustrates the digestion of fat and storage of fat. High fat diets will create mushroomed fat storage cells.

THE BODY AND FAT

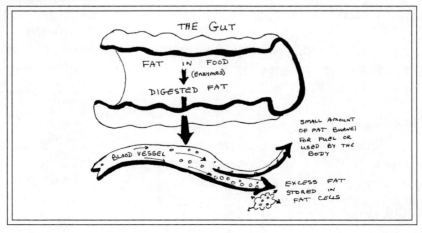

DO WE NEED FAT?

The body needs a small amount of fat for health. Although we can manufacture most fatty components within our cells, including cholesterol, we do need *one tablespoon of vegetable fat* (oil) per day. That's all! That amounts to 3–5% of our total food energy per day. One tablespoon of vegetable oil contains 125 calories of energy and is pure fat. The body does not really need any fat from animal sources. It thrives on vegetable fat alone. However, a small amount of animal fat is acceptable.

THE TYPES OF FAT

Monounsaturated Fat:
   olive, canola, peanut oil
Polyunsaturated Fat:
   Safflower, sunflower, soybean, cottonseed and
   sesame oil
Saturated Fat:
   Butter, lard, shortening, meat fats, poultry fats,
   dairy products, coconut and palm oil.

THE GOOD, THE BAD, THE UGLY

All fats are high in calories (9 calories/gram)!

Monounsaturated fats are the "good fats." They help to lower bad cholesterol and are excellent products for cooking and baking. Polyunsaturated fats, also "good fats," are present in vegetable oils. Good vegetable oils are a mixture of monounsaturated and polyunsaturated fats. Vegetable oils make food moist, and enhance the flavor of foods.

Saturated fats are the "bad fats" in the sights of the nutritionist sharpshooter! Many of us can remember the days when it was normal to cook fish in butter! The American Heart Association and the Canadian food guide recommend that saturated fat comprise less than 10% of daily calories. Saturated fat, with its high calories (9 calories/gram) and tendency to plug arteries in the human body, is the main cause of high cholesterol.

What is the "ugly fat"? It's the fat we put on around our waists and hips from eating too much fat! Unless we reduce excess fat in food, 50% of us will develop fat related disease before the age of 65.

WHAT HAPPENS TO EXTRA FAT IN OUR DIETS?

Extra fat will be stored in our fat cells. These jolly little guys will simply get plumper. Our bodies, somehow genetically programmed for impending famine, won't waste fat. We save it until we can use the energy. Extra fat stores in our fat cells can be metabolized to glucose (sugar) during prolonged exercise. After 20 minutes of exercise our bodies begin to mix fat with glucose as fuel.

THE BEST COOKING OILS

The best oil for cooking or baking should have: high monounsaturated fat, less polyunsaturated fat and very little saturated fat. Olive oil fits that description. It is the best vegetable oil. It is followed in merit by canola oil and safflower oil. Recently, nutty and sweet oils made from almond, avocado and hazelnuts have appeared. These are healthy products that bring interesting flavors to foods, especially stir-fries.

Tub (semi-solid) margarine is the best vegetable spread. Choose a margarine with low saturated fat. *Light* margarines replace fat with air by whipping the margarine, or replace fat with water.

HYDROGENATION OF VEGETABLE FATS

Hydrogenation changes unsaturated fat into a type of saturated fat. This process is used by food producers to make liquid vegetable oils more solid (e.g... margarine) and to improve the shelf life of products such as cereals, cookies and crackers. Unfortunately, this process creates *trans-fatty acid* which behaves like saturated fat in the body. Read labels carefully to avoid saturated and hydrogenated fats. If you cook with a margarine rather than a good cooking oil (such as olive oil or canola oil) select a product made from a healthy vegetable oil (canola, safflower, sunflower) and avoid hydrogenated vegetable fat.

KEYS TO REDUCING FAT INTAKE

- Reduce meat portions. Take more vegetables, pasta, potatoes or rice.
- Remove all visible fat and skin from meat before cooking.
- Reduce the use of fats and oils in cooking. Use a non-stick frying pan with vegetable oil cooking spray or broth for stir fries or sautés. Use onions, garlic, herbs and spices for flavor.
- Barbecue, broil, microwave or roast with a drip pan. Avoid frying with oil or butter.
- Read the labels to choose foods with good fat (mono and polyunsaturated).
- If you enjoy fish, eat it frequently.

OMEGA–3 OILS: FISH OILS

Fish oils contain polyunsaturated fats called omega–3 fatty acids. These fats have been shown to lower bad cholesterol and protect us from heart disease. Fish oils also have promise in treating rheumatoid arthritis.

THE FINAL DIET AND FAT

Give the body fat and it will become just that. To burn fat, we must exercise. To lose weight, we must exercise and restrict fat in our diets.

The Final Diet will teach you how to prepare and enjoy scrumptious low fat meals while rediscovering normal weight and invigorating fitness.

PROTEIN: PROSE ABOUT PROTEIN

The body needs protein. Our bodies are able to construct thousands of different protein products. Proteins in the body fight infection, build muscle and serve as enzymes for chemical reactions.

Food proteins are attacked by digestive enzymes in the gut. They are broken to protein components called amino acids. These amino acids pass through the gut wall and into the blood stream. They are delivered to the liver and the muscle. The liver is a factory for building new proteins for the body. The muscles use amino acids to repair damaged muscle proteins. See how the body absorbs and uses protein:

THE BODY AND PROTEIN

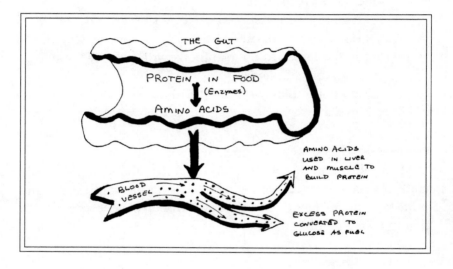

HOW MUCH PROTEIN DO I NEED?

The human body needs 16% of its calories as protein. For a 150 pound person this is 70 grams or 280 calories of protein per day. Most north Americans eat twice that amount! The problem with too much protein is the company it keeps. Most animal sources of protein (e.g. Meat, milk, eggs) also contain large amounts of fat. For example, four ounces of lean grilled hamburger contain 32 grams (128 calories) of protein with 24 grams (216 calories) of fat. The extra protein can be converted to glucose and burned as fuel, but the body prefers simple sources of fuel–carbohydrates (rice, potatoes, bread, pasta, vegetables, fruit).

Eating extra protein will not cause us to suddenly sprout large biceps ala Schwartzenegger. The only way large muscles bulge is with large work! Heavy muscular activity will need extra protein for muscle repair and new muscle formation.

EXCESS PROTEIN-HARMFUL

Large amounts of protein will harm our bodies because of the excess fat that travels with animal proteins. Excess protein use is harmful in a global sense. Animal proteins are the top of the food chain. The milk or chicken or pork we consume is the result of feeding vegetable protein (grains) to domestic animals. The process is expensive and detrimental to the environment (animal waste, carcasses, methane gas).

In 1990, 70% of our food protein came from animal sources. In 1900, 70% of our ancestor's food protein came from vegetable sources. High fat animal proteins have factored strongly in the modern plague of obesity. Good sources of vegetable proteins exist in beans, peas, lentils and grains. They are cheap and low in fat.

LOW FAT SOURCES OF PROTEIN

Low fat sources of animal protein are turkey, chicken, fish, skim milk, egg whites, 1% cottage cheese, no fat yogurt and ultra-lean red meats. It is difficult to get adequate protein from vegetable protein alone (vegetarianism). Care is needed to combine foods correctly to supply the body with the necessary amino acids. Vegetarian foods plus eggs, dairy products, fish and/or poultry create a fulfilling diet that meets protein needs.

THE FINAL DIET AND PROTEIN

The Final Diet uses vegetable and low fat animal protein to fill the body's needs. High fat and high calorie protein sources are avoided to encourage good health and promote weight loss.

CARBOHYDRATES: A CHORUS!

History will show that Adam and Eve ate well. They enjoyed carbohydrates–natural human food.

Carbohydrates, in all shapes and sizes, are long or short chains of sugar molecules. In the gut, all carbohydrates (except fiber) are broken down by enzymes to glucose molecules. The glucose migrates through the gut wall into the blood stream–as high octane cell fuel. *Glucose is the body's only cell fuel.*

Athletes eat pasta (carbohydrate) before their tests of skill and strength rather than steak (protein and fat). Pasta is rapidly digested to glucose, a ready source of fuel during the match, not three hours later.

Excess glucose in the blood is tacked together into chains to form glycogen in the liver and muscle. This important carbohydrate is stored, ready to provide energy for quick release during times of stress or during exercise. The body normally stores 500 grams of glycogen with about 2 liters (4 pounds) of water in the body. Starvation diets, which burn glycogen first, cause rapid initial weight loss when glycogen is burned. The storage water leaves the body as urine. Unfortunately, all the weight quickly returns when the starvation is over and when the body rehydrates.

The diagram on the opposite page illustrates how carbohydrates are absorbed and used by the body.

THE BODY AND CARBOHYDRATE

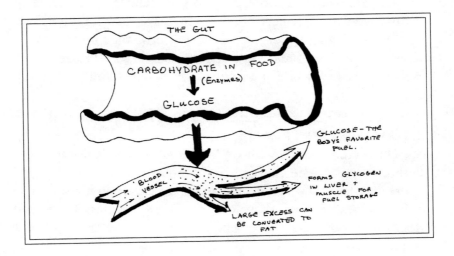

TYPES OF CARBOHYDRATE

Simple sugars such as glucose, sucrose and fructose are simple carbohydrates. They are found in sweet foods (sugar, fruit, juices, honey).

Starch and cellulose are long chain complex carbohydrates. Starch is found in potatoes, cereals and vegetables. Indigestible cellulose is found in plant products such as pea pods and corn cobs. Indigestible carbohydrates, which pass right through the gut, are called *fibre* in foods. Bran, the casings of the germ from grains, is a good example of a fiber food.

Carbohydrate foods are complex if they contain mostly long chain carbohydrates. The common complex carbohydrate foods are rice, potatoes, grain products (bread, cereals), pasta, beans, vegetables and fruit.

FIBRE: WHY IS IT HEALTHY?

High fiber foods such as vegetables, bran cereals, fruits and whole wheat bread are an excellent source of bulk in the diet. The indigestible fiber swells with water in the gut and promotes rapid passage of a soft mushy stool! (We won't get more graphic).

In African societies, where high fiber, low fat diets prevail, food passes through the gut in under 24 hours. In our constipated, low carbohydrate, high fat society, bowel transit time is often three to four days. Interestingly, bowel cancer is very rare in African society. Japanese people, who take a low fat, high fiber diet, have a much lower rate of heart disease than north Americans. There is impressive evidence that high fiber in foods reduces obesity while improving bowel habit and preventing disease.

THE RIGHT AMOUNT OF THE RIGHT STUFF

Our bodies thrive with 60% of more of our calories from carbohydrate. Since glucose is the body's chosen fuel, good sense dictates that we feed it glucose chains (carbohydrates). The free water stored in many carbohydrates such as fruits and vegetables contains the essential vitamins and minerals our bodies crave.

THERMOGENESIS: THE SECRET IS OUT

Scientists have discovered a surprising fact about the way we digest complex carbohydrates. The body uses or burns about 10% of the calories in carbohydrates in the process of digestion! This consumption of calories is called thermogenesis. While digesting, the body produces and releases heat. An 80 calorie apple requires 8 calories of energy to be eaten! This explains the pleasant warmth we feel after a meal of pasta and bread.

Thermogenesis gives carbohydrate foods a 10% calorie discount.

CONVERTING CARBOHYDRATES TO FAT

The first task the body will perform, if offered excess carbohydrate, is to fill the body's glycogen stores (500 grams). Since glycogen is stored 4 parts water to 1 part glycogen, we often gain a few pounds with a high carbohydrate meal. This weight gain is not fat!

The body can convert excess carbohydrate to fat. Only about 25% of extra carbohydrate will follow that path. The body is reluctant to do the complex chemical steps needed to convert carbohydrate to fat.

THE FINAL DIET AND CARBOHYDRATE

Reducing fat and increasing complex carbohydrates are the two pillars of the Final Diet. The two principles work together to reduce calories, to reduce harmful fats and to give to give the body the complex carbohydrates it cherishes.

ALCOHOL

Alcohol has eroded a special niche in the bedrock of nutrition. Alcohol has 7 calories/gram versus 9 calories/gram for fat and 4 calories/gram for carbohydrate and protein. Alcohol is absorbed rapidly without digestion through the gut wall. In excess of 2 oz. of hard alcohol or 2 beers per day, damages the liver and the heart. Alcohol, in excess, causes enormous poverty, suffering and health care expenses. The final diet suggests no more than 1 light beer or 4 oz. of light wine per day.

WHAT FOOD DOES MY BODY WANT AND NEED?

The following chart shows how the typical north American diet compares with the body's basic needs and with the *Final Diet.*

	% CALORIES FAT	% CALORIES PROTEIN	% CALORIES CARBOHYDRATE
Typical North American diet	40%	25%	35%
My body's needs	5%	15%	60% or more
The FINAL DIET	15-20%	15-20%	60% or more

THE FINAL DIET ALLOWS

- Enough fat (15–20% of calories) to make food interesting and palatable but little enough to reduce the calories and the harmful effects.
- An ideal protein intake (15–20% of calories) to ensure healthy muscles and proteins.

- The rest of the daily calories are filled with healthy, wholesome complex and simple carbohydrates–the body's natural food.

Why most diets fail–three scenarios

Scenario one: The 'starvation' trap (too few calories)

George is 30 years old, 5'10" and weighs 210 pounds. He has a medium frame. His ideal weight is 165 lbs (chapter 4). He has gained 45 pounds over 10 years as he stopped competitive running and started work as a traveling salesman. Restaurant meals are a great convenience on the road. 40% of his calories are from fat in foods. George knows nothing about nutrition. He wouldn't recognize a saturated fat if it honked at him.

George attempts to lose his weight in 3 months. A commercial high protein, low carbohydrate diet franchise recommends a 1200 calorie starvation diet. He starts a diet that would not keep a 90 pound pygmy happy. The body starves under 1200 calories a day.

George's body first attacks glycogen (strings of glucose) stored in his liver and muscle. Since glycogen is stored 4:1 with water, George's body loses 4 pounds, mostly water, in 3 days. He's dehydrated, but happy!

Because George's body is starving, it burns muscle protein and fat from fat cells. The result of the body consuming itself is release of toxic chemicals into the circulation—ketones. Ketones create a feeling of achiness, fatigue, lethargy and headache and give a sweet, odor to his breath. George is now beginning to feel like a starving Ethiopian—tired, dehydrated, light-headed—no energy to work or play. When he exerts himself his blood sugar drops. He feels like fainting.

George thinks, "I'd rather die fat than live like this." However, he's paid good money to feel this bad. He persists. By the second week, George has lost 10 pounds but he feels and looks like death. His body realizes that George no longer loves it, and slows his metabolism! By week 3 he has lost 14 pounds—some water, some valuable muscle and some fat. His body has adjusted to starvation and plateaus—he stops losing weight for a whole week!

Disgusted, George tears up his membership card, walks slowly (due to dizziness) to his car and drives to the nearest "burger joint" for real food.

George has not learned anything about food. He is not exercising. He has no new life-style to replace the old ways that made him heavy. Sadly, George quickly returns to his old ways. He regains his 'lost weight'. He is left with four scars: a slower metabolism, a reduction of his muscle mass, an experience of failure and a much lighter wallet.

THE LESSON:

Starvation (high protein, low carbohydrate) diets (1200 calories or less) don't work as a *permanent* positive life style and weight loss tool. Diets that don't respect the body's needs are doomed.

SCENARIO TWO: THE 'TINY PORTION' TRAP

Sally is 42 years old, 5'4" and 160 pounds. She has battled obesity all her adult life. Her ideal weight is 120 pounds on a small frame (chapter 4).

Her plan of attack for January 1 is as old as the calendar. She skips breakfast, has a tiny lunch and a light supper. She is convinced that *all food is bad* and that her metabolism is so slow that she must deprive herself to be slim.

For the first week she does well. By 2 P.M. She is ready to eat her sneakers—but she hangs in. She drools as she watches her family eat pie and ice cream. She finds herself sniffing donut boxes. She dreams about deep fried chicken.

By week three she has lost 6 pounds, but her personality has changed. She thinks constantly about food. She is irritable and angry. She refuses to cook meals for her family. If she can't eat it—why cook it? While she slowly loses weight, her poor teenagers gain weight at fast food joints.

At the end of week four she has 2 chocolate donuts as a treat…then a giant hamburger, and so on…

The lesson:

Food deprivation creates preoccupation with food. It does not change habits. It does not allow people to satisfy their hunger with alternative low fat, high carbohydrate foods while allowing weight loss.

Scenario three: The 'wrong food' trap

Phillip is 52 years old, 5'8" and 190 pounds. He has a small frame with an ideal weight of 140 pounds. He has a sedentary job. He loves meat! At a cocktail party, Phillip chats with an old friend, Paul, who is slim and athletic. Curious for his friend's secret, Phillip asks what type of meals he eats. The friend replies "I like meat, good lean red meat! And lots of potatoes and veggies and salads."

Phillip heard *meat*, particularly *red meat*. He fails to discover that Paul swims five times per week and works hard to minimize fat in other foods. Phillip fails to gather the true secrets of Paul's good looks.

Phillip's diet flops, as expected. He eats far too much fatty meat (at 9 calories/gram). He eats it with french fries and other fatty foods. After two months his weight creeps to 200 pounds. He is unaware that his cholesterol was *high*, and now is very high. He cuts down on bread, pasta, rice and cereals (good carbohydrates) to cut out "starch." He continues to eat 6–8 oz. of meat every day. Eventually, the idea of weight loss is forgotten. Phillip becomes one of the "happy" obese people who have abandoned hope.

At 58, Phillip drops dead of a heart attack while playing golf. The fat deposits in his coronary arteries, the blood vessels that give fresh blood to the heart muscle, are completely blocked. The heart muscle quits! Phillip's diet has contributed to his untimely death.

The lesson:

High fat foods in medium to large portions make weight loss impossible, and expose us to serious health risks.

THE FINAL DIET: DARE TO DREAM

- We will set a reasonable body weight goal to achieve in a rational time frame (be patient!).
- We will feed our *ideal body*, not our overweight body. As we visualize our ideal body, our present body will slowly conform to that model.
- We will enjoy ample delicious low fat, high carbohydrate meals. We won't be hungry.
- We will exercise to preserve our muscle protein and help our bodies burn off stored fat.
- By treating our bodies like our ideal leaner, fitter bodies, the Final Diet will help us make that transformation.

A SUMMARY OF CHAPTER TWO:

HOW THE BODY USES FOOD

1. All food is composed of a mixture of Fat, Protein, and Carbohydrate.

2. The Fat component of food has 225% of the calories found in the protein or carbohydrate components (The 9 to 4 rule)

3. Eating Fat makes us fat.

4. Animal fats (saturated) are harmful. Vegetable fats (monounsaturated, polyunsaturated) are beneficial, in limited amounts.

5. Protein foods in excess of our body's *needs* are of no benefit. Animal protein is often high in saturated fat.

6. Carbohydrates, especially complex carbohydrates— pasta, rice, potatoes, beans, grain products, vegetables and fruit—are the body's favorite foods.

7. Reducing fat intake and increasing complex carbohy- drate intake (the Final Diet) will result in normal weight and vibrant health.

The Final Diet will help us maintain a lean, fit body...

FOR LIFE!

CHAPTER 3

TWO INGREDIENTS FOR SUCCESS

To achieve and maintain a fit and slim body, we must stress two vital ingredients before we teach you *"The Final Diet."*

You must have the support of your family and/or a close friend.

My wife and children and I have made *"The Final Diet"* a dynamic family event. We frequently talk about carbohydrate, fat and exercise. We read about nutrition and fitness and teach each other secrets. Planning and preparation of interesting and delicious low fat meals has become an enjoyable part of our family life.

Do not impose a "new diet" on your family or spouse without their understanding and support. Share the "fat revolution" with your family or seek a close friend who wants to lose weight. You need at least one teammate. You will appreciate the support and the sharing of your success.

Regular exercise at least four times a week is necessary with "The Final Diet."

The human body is part of the natural kingdom. To maintain

the protein stores that make up muscle, you must use muscle, especially during periods when you are dropping back to ideal body weight. Also, exercise is a great way to increase the body's use of food calories!

Don't worry—we're not asking you to become the incredible hulk. Forty minutes of pleasant, vigorous walking, jogging, biking or the equivalent is exactly what your body needs. See "exercise—the second essential", chapter 11 for a full exercise prescription.

Note:

All diabetics should consult a Dietitian or a Physician before starting a high complex carbohydrate diet.

CHAPTER 4

THE FINAL DIET 'GAME PLAN'

In this chapter we will assist you to set goals for your new low fat diet that will help you achieve your ideal weight with *no hunger or pain.*

THE FAT UNIT

To make fat control even more simple, we will introduce the *"fat unit."* A fat unit is the same as a gram of fat in food.

1 fat unit = 1 gram of fat = 9 calories of fat energy

IDEAL WEIGHT AND FAT INTAKE

Now we will help you find your ideal weight and discover how many fat units (fat grams) you should choose as your limit per day. We suggest that you hold fat intake to 15–20% of your diet. Remember, your body *needs* only about 3–5% of its calories as vegetable fat. As you reduce fat intake to under 20% your body weight will fall.

DO I HAVE TO COUNT CALORIES?

The key to weight loss on *"The Final Diet"* is to replace fatty foods with healthy high carbohydrate foods (9 calories/gram to 4 calories/gram).

1.   For the *first two weeks* we suggest that you keep track of total *calories and fat units* in your daily food intake. A great way to do this is to follow our delicious and nutritious meal plans (chapter 15).

2.   *After two weeks* on *"The Final Diet"* you should keep only a rough idea of calories. You don't want to feel obsessed by calories! Carefully count the fat units in your food to keep within your daily fat unit goal. Achieve your fat unit goal and you will achieve and maintain your ideal weight.

3.   *By the end of 4–6 weeks* you will have a good command of how many fat units are in the foods you eat regularly and will have mastered the simple food choices to avoid foods with high fat content (see smart substitutions, chapter 9). You will no longer need to count fat units.

The Final Diet: Step One

FINDING IDEAL WEIGHT

Although none of us should be obsessed with ideal weight, it is good to set a reasonable weight goal as we start this positive life-style change. Table 4a will help you find a reasonable weight goal.

Large frame or small frame?
If you are not sure if you have a large frame, do this: circle your wrist with your thumb and middle finger. If they overlap—you're small. If they don't meet—you're large. If they just touch—take the mid point in the range for your height as your ideal weight.
If you are over 30 pounds over your ideal weight, pick the large frame ideal weight as your initial weight goal. You can lower it later! We'll help you learn to eat the right foods in the perfect amounts for your ideal body.

Table 4a (adapted from Health & Welfare Canada Body Mass Index Data)

WOMEN					MEN			
HEIGHT		IDEAL WEIGHT			HEIGHT		IDEAL WEIGHT	
FEET/INCHES	CM	SMALL FRAME	LARGE FRAME		FEET/INCHES	CM	SMALL FRAME	LARGE FRAME
4' 10"	148	98	120		5' 0"	152	110	130
4' 11"	150	100	125		5' 1"	155	115	135
5' 0"	152	105	128		5' 2"	157	120	140
5' 1"	155	108	132		5' 3"	160	123	145
5' 2"	157	112	135		5' 4"	163	126	150
5' 3"	160	115	138		5' 5"	165	130	155
5' 4"	163	118	142		5' 6"	168	133	160
5' 5"	165	122	148		5' 7"	170	136	165
5' 6"	168	125	150		5' 8"	173	140	170
5' 7"	170	130	153		5' 9"	175	145	174
5' 8"	173	135	158		5' 10"	178	150	180
5' 9"	175	140	163		5' 11"	180	155	185
5' 10"	178	143	168		6' 0"	183	158	190
5' 11"	180	148	173		6' 1"	186	162	195
6' 0"	183	155	180		6' 2"	188	165	200
6' 1"	186	160	185		6' 3"	191	170	205

My height is:_____

My ideal weight is:_____

The Final Diet: Step Two finding daily calorie limit and fat unit goals

We will now set our calorie limit. Women should consult table 4b and men should consult table 4c (next two pages)

On the Final Diet we will take 15–20% of our food calories in the form of fat calories. The tables 4b (women) and 4c (men) will help us to pick out a range of fat units that establish that goal.

Example:

Samantha is 5'8" with a medium frame.
Her ideal weight is 147 pounds (table 4a)

She looks at table 4b under 147 pounds. Samantha's calorie limit per day is 1650 calories on *The Final Diet*. If she took 15% of those calories as fat she would take 250 fat calories. If she takes 20% of her calories as fat she would take 340 fat calories. The Final Diet suggests that she set her daily fat goal in the 250 to 340 calorie range. Since 9 calories of fat come from 1 gram of fat or 1 fat unit, her fat goal per day is 28–38 fat grams or fat units per day. Table 4b has already done the math for her. For the sake of simplicity, Samantha could remember 35 fat units as her daily fat goal as it sits comfortably in the 15–20% fat unit range for Samantha's ideal weight. If she finds 35 fat units plenty, she could move her fat goal down to 28 or 30 fat units per day to promote more rapid weight loss.

Men can find their daily calorie limits and fat goals in table 4c.

Table 4b

WOMEN					
IDEAL BODY WEIGHT (POUNDS)	CALORIE LIMIT PER DAY	FAT CALORIES		FAT UNITS	
		20%	15%	20%	15%
95	1100	220	170	24	18
100	1150	230	175	25	19
105	1250	245	185	27	20
110	1300	255	195	28	21
115	1350	270	200	30	22
120	1400	280	210	31	23
125	1450	290	220	32	24
130	1500	305	230	34	25
135	1550	315	235	35	26
140	1600	330	245	37	27
145	1650	340	250	38	28
150	1700	350	260	39	29
155	1800	360	270	40	30
160	1850	375	280	42	31
165	1900	385	290	43	32
170	2000	400	300	44	33
175	2050	410	310	46	34
180	2100	420	320	47	35
185	2200	435	330	48	36

STEP TWO: WOMEN

My *ideal body weight* is_____ pounds.
My *ideal calorie limit per day* is_____ calories.
My *fat unit goal at 20%* is_____ units.
My *fat unit goal at 15%* is_____ units.

1 fat unit = 1 gram of fat = 9 calories of energy

Table 4c

MEN					
IDEAL BODY WEIGHT (POUNDS)	**CALORIE LIMIT PER DAY**	**FAT CALORIES**		**FAT UNITS**	
		20%	**15%**	**20%**	**15%**
110	1450	290	220	32	24
115	1500	300	225	33	25
120	1550	310	230	34	26
125	1600	320	240	36	27
130	1700	340	250	38	28
135	1750	350	260	39	29
140	1800	360	270	40	30
145	1900	380	280	42	31
150	1950	390	290	43	32
155	2000	400	300	45	34
160	2100	420	310	47	35
165	2150	430	320	48	36
170	2200	440	330	49	37
175	2300	460	340	51	38
180	2350	470	350	52	39
185	2400	480	360	53	40
190	2450	490	370	54	41
195	2550	510	380	57	42
200	2600	520	390	58	43
205	2650	530	400	59	44

STEP TWO: MEN

My *ideal body weight* is_____ pounds.
My *ideal calorie limit per day* is_____ calories.
My *fat unit goal at 20%* is_____ units.
My *fat unit goal at 15%* is_____ units.

1 fat unit = 1 gram of fat = 9 calories of energy

Congratulations, you have now set *"Final Diet"* goals that will allow you to steadily drop your weight to your ideal weight.

FOUR RULES:

1. *Be patient!* It took years to put the baggage on…expect that you will take weeks to months to shed it. The goals you have set will cause 1–2 pounds of weight loss per week. You will lose more if you increase your exercise! The authors lost weight at 2–3 pounds per week to reach their ideal weights (Mike—54 lbs. in 20 weeks and Linda—15 lbs. in 8 weeks).

2. Weigh yourself *once a week* on the same scale, ideally in the morning, in the buff..

3. *Exercise at least 4 times per week*. It prevents muscle loss during weight loss *and* it burns calories to speed weight loss (Chapter 11; Exercise—the Second Essential).

4. As you learn about food and begin to enjoy low fat food, *The Final Diet will become a new food habit that promotes health and vigor*. Don't rush—*take time to change your approach to food.*

NATURE'S RULE	
3500 CALORIES EXTRA FOOD or **LESS EXERCISE**	**1 POUND GAIN**
3500 CALORIES LESS FOOD or **MORE EXERCISE**	**1 POUND LOSS**

A REVIEW

My *ideal body weight* is_____ pounds.
My *ideal calorie limit per day* is_____ calories.
My *initial (20%) fat unit goal at* is_____ fat units.
My *ultimate (15%) fat unit goal at* is_____ fat units.

AN EXAMPLE:
HOW BONNIE BEAT THE BULGE WITH THE FINAL DIET (WITHOUT STARVATION!)

Bonnie is 5'6" with a medium build. She is a 42 year old working mother who now weighs 165 pounds.

Her *ideal body weight* is 140 pounds (table 4a)

Her *calorie goal per day* is 1600 calories (table 4b)

Her *fat unit goal* is 27 (15%) to 37 (20%) (table 4b)

On the next page, see how Bonnie substituted low fat foods for high fat foods on *The Final Diet*.

She cut her daily calories from 2450 to 1490 for the day. She reduced her fat intake from 130 fat units (fat grams) or 9 x 130 = 1170 calories to 22 fat units (fat grams) or 9 x 22 = 198 calories. Cutting fat greatly reduces the daily totals for both calorie and fat. She finished her day *below* her calorie and fat unit goal.

In spite of large reductions in calories and fat units, Bonnie ate excellent meals on *The Final Diet*. She was *not* hungry. On the Final diet you can eat well—no starvation.

---

1 Fat Unit = 1 Gram of Fat = 9 Calories

BEFORE				THE FINAL DIET		
FOOD	CAL.	FAT UNITS		FOOD	CAL.	FAT UNITS
BREAKFAST:				BREAKFAST:		
1 egg	80	6		3/4 cup Raisin Bran	130	1
2 toast	140	2		1 cup skim milk	86	0
1 tbsp. margarine	100	7		1 cup strawberries	45	1
1 tbsp. jam	55	0		1 piece raisin toast	70	1
1 cup 2% milk	120	5		1 tbsp. lite jam	20	0
coffee	0	0		coffee	0	0
TOTAL	495	20			350	3
				TOTAL		
SNACK:				SNACK:		
carrot muffin	260	14		1/2 cup no-fat yogurt with	100	0
coffee	0	0		blueberries		
				coffee	0	0
TOTAL	260	14		TOTAL	100	0
LUNCH:				LUNCH:		
2 oz. lean ham on 2 slices of	80	3		1 1/2 cups tuna, celery and	150	0
rye bread	140	0		grape salad (recipe page 123)		
1 tbsp. margarine	100	7		1 apple	80	0
1 tbsp. mayonnaise	100	7		diet drink	1	0
3 chocolate chip cookies	150	7				
black tea	0	0				
TOTAL	570	24		TOTAL	231	0
SNACK:				SNACK:		
nothing				8 oz. hot chocolate (light)	45	0
SUPPER:				SUPPER:		
4 oz. deep fried haddock in	240	10		1 1/2 cups linguini	300	2
batter				9 large sauteed shrimp in	75	1
2 tbsp. tartar sauce	160	18		1 cup green bean stirfry with	44	0
medium baked potato	120	0		1 tbsp. olive oil	120	13
2 tbsp. sour cream	50	5		1 1/2 cups green salad	50	0
3/4 cup coleslaw	10	0		1 tbsp. no-fat dressing	15	0
2 tbsp. mayonnaise	200	22				
1/2 cup creamed corn	95	1				
TOTAL	875	56		TOTAL	604	16
DESSERT:				DESSERT:		
nothing				1/2 cantaloupe	50	0
				3.5 oz. blackcherry frozen	110	3
				yogurt		
				TOTAL	160	3
SNACK:						
25 potato chips	250	16				
TOTALS FOR THE DAY	2450	130		TOTALS FOR THE DAY	1490	22

What did Bonnie change?

Before starting the "final diet" Bonnie felt she was careful with food (2% milk, no cream or sugar in her coffee, 'healthy' muffins, skipping dessert). She tried to choose healthy foods (fish, potatoes, lean ham). However, by feeding herself 2450 calories of *high fat (48% of her calories were from fat!!)* foods, she provided the right amount of food to keep the bulges *on* her 165 pound body.

The final diet helps her eliminate the "fat traps" (regular margarine, regular mayonnaise, cookies, muffins, sauces, creams and junk food!). By making healthy, low–fat choices, Bonnie reduces her calories for the day by 40% and her fat units by 80%. She remains well below her calorie goal and her fat unit goal for the day. She eats well. She could have an extra snack of 4 cups of air popped popcorn (calories 90, fat units 2) if she feels hungry toward bedtime.

Bonnie starts a brisk walking program 5 days a week (2 miles to work, 2 miles home).

As she meets her food goals and enjoys her brisk daily walk, she will lose 2–3 pounds/week on "The Final Diet."

Special Times:

• Pregnancy: the "Final Diet" in pregnancy?

Yes, but ask your dietitian, family doctor or obstetrician for a *daily calorie goal* to use in table 4b. Follow the 20% fat unit goal. You should *gain* 20–25 pounds with pregnancy! Take 3 to 4 servings of milk per day.

• Children: the "Final "Diet" for children?

Yes, children over 10 can follow the "Final Diet." Under 16, obtain a daily calorie goal from your dietitian or family doctor to plug into table 4b or 4c to ensure that your child is not deprived of calories during a time of body growth. *"The Final Diet"* is nutritionally sound. Increase milk to 3–4 glasses/day.

• BREAST FEEDING: THE "FINAL DIET" AND BREAST FEEDING?

We would suggest that you increase fat consumption to about 25–30% of total calories while breast feeding. Ask your dietitian, family doctor or pediatrician for a calorie goal while breast feeding and increase milk to 3–4 glasses/day.

Chapter 5

Great Foods—Part 1:
The Complex Carbohydrates—
the Stuff of Life

The Super Seven

1. Grain products (bread, cereals)
2. Potatoes
3. Rice
4. Pasta
5. Beans
6. Veggies
7. Fruit

The complex carbohydrates are the great foods that provide over 60% of our calories on *The Final Diet*. They make us slim as we enjoy their benefits.

With the advent of 'fast foods' and high fat, high protein diets in the 1950s, the complex carbohydrate fell out of favor–as "peasant food." The result was "widespread" obesity and the health hazards of high fat.

Complex carbohydrates are full of riches

Complex carbohydrates satisfy most of the body's nutritional needs. Starches and sugars provide vital glucose for *fuel*. Fibre provides *bulk* in foods. Vegetable proteins are used for *building* cells. Essential *nutrients*—calcium, iron, magnesium, phosphorous, potassium, zinc and others—and *vitamins* A, B, C, and E are provided in abundance. Almost all of the fibre and nutrients in complex carbohydrates are in the coatings—the bran of grains and rice and the skins of fruits and veggies. Don't throw away the best part! The only essential nutrient or vitamin that we need from animal sources is vitamin B12—complex carbohydrates provide the rest.

THE SUPER SEVEN: COMPLEX CARBOHYDRATES

1. GRAIN PRODUCTS

Since antiquity, bread has been called "the staff of life." What do most of us do when we get obese and want to lose weight? *We stop eating bread—a wrong move!* Bread is nutritious and delicious—low in calories and filling. It contains valuable protein, vitamins and nutrients. It is low in fat and high in fibre. It fills the stomach up, and is excellent for the bowel (You'll be as regular as taxation notices!).

A. BREAD PRODUCTS:

Below we show some vital statistics about common bread products.

PRODUCT	CALORIES	PROTEIN (gm)	FAT UNITS	FIBRE (gm)
Homemade honey whole wheat raisin bread (medium slice). (Recipe pg. 95)	110	5	1	7
Whole wheat pita pocket	106	4	.5	4
White bread (1/2" slice)	70	2.6	1	0
Light whole wheat bread (1/2" slice)	60	2.4	1	2

THE BEST BREADS

- Homemade low-fat whole wheat bread. This is wonderful, healthy bread—we bake this at our house every 1–2 days (see recipe pg. 95).
- Any whole wheat store-bought bread. Bread made from refined white or dark flour (even enriched!) has little fibre and is reduced in protein, nutrients and vitamins. When we buy bread, we check the label–it should state "whole wheat" and the fibre content should be over 2 grams per ½" slice. We know that we are getting the best.
- There are "light" whole wheat breads with as few as 40 calories/slice.

Forget: Bread = Starch = Fattening!
Learn: Bread = Healthy Fiber, Fuel, Protein, Nutrients &
Vitamins

It's what you put on bread that counts! See chapter 8, problem 3, to avoid the *"great bread/bad spread"* problem.

B. FLOUR

We don't have to be brain surgeons to realize that flour is important in nutrition.

TYPE	CALORIES/CUP	GOOD/BAD
WHOLE WHEAT FLOUR	400	**THE BEST.** Retains the fibre, protein, nutrients and vitamins of grain.
ALL PURPOSE "ENRICHED" FLOUR	500	**NOT SO GOOD.** Higher in calories and lower in everything our bodies want and need.

Wheat (the grain) contains most essential human nutrients, primarily in the bran coat of the central germ. The process of refining grain to all purpose white flour removes most of the valuable bran and germ. Whole wheat flour retains almost all of the "goodies." It's better if it is prepared in a "stone ground" fashion. *Bake with whole wheat flour!*

C. CEREALS

Excellent cereals contain the best parts—bran and germ—of the grain. Look for cereals that are high in fibre, low in fat and low in calories! A good cereal will have 4–5 grams of fibre per 3/4 cup serving.

SOME EXCELLENT BREAKFAST CEREALS:

GRAIN:	CEREAL:
Wheat	Shredded Wheat, Puffed Wheat, Total Bran Flakes, Raisin Bran
Corn	Nutri-Grain, Corn Flakes, Corn Bran
Rolled Oats	Rolled Oats (not instant), Cheerios

Many cereals (e.g. Frosted Flakes) are high in added sugar and low in fibre and should be avoided. Granola cereals are generally "pseudo health foods"—high in calories and fat and moderate in fibre. The recommended portion (½ cup) wouldn't satisfy a 4 year old. *Read the labels on cereal boxes.*

2. POTATOES

What else do most people do when they want to lose weight?— *They stop eating potatoes. Another wrong move!*

The potato, about 80% water, has valuable fibre, protein, iodine and other nutrients and vitamins. Many of the nutrients are in the skin. For 5 delicious potato recipes see the potato recipe section (pages 151-155). As you can see, a large order of french fries (100 calories potato / 370 calories fat!) fills the fat need for *"The Final Diet"* for a day.

THE GLORIOUS POTATO

POTATO	CALORIES	PROTEIN (g)	FAT UNITS
(5 oz) Baked Potato with skin	160	3.5	0
(5 oz) Potato (boiled - no skin)	120	3	0
(5 oz) Baked Potato with 2 tbsp. no-fat yogurt, chives, pepper, garlic	188	6	0
(5 oz) Baked Potato with 1 tsp. butter 2 tbsp. sour cream	160 36 52 248	4	0 4 5 9
(5 oz) 30 French Fries	370	6	25

3. RICE

Rice is the most important staple for the *thin* half of the world. Brown rice—with bran coating and germ—is an excellent source of vitamins, minerals, protein and fibre. Polished or white rice is primarily starch (big chains of sugar). Unfortunately, much of the third world insists on polished rice. Discarding the most nutritious part of the rice results in protein deficiency (kwashiorkor) and vitamin deficiency (especially vitamin B1 deficiency—beri-beri). Over 95% of the rice sold in the U.S. is white, polished rice.

Buy Brown Rice!!

You will prefer the slightly nutty, richer taste compared to bland white rice. If you want white rice, choose the parboiled, enriched rice which is processed to keep nutrients.

RICE	CALORIES	PROTEIN	FAT UNITS
Brown - 1 cup cooked	230	5 grams	1
White (enriched parboiled) - 1 cup	185	3.7 grams	0

Try the great stir-fry recipes served with rice (or pasta) in the meat and poultry recipe sections of chapter 16. Also, try rice pudding for a nutritious and tasty dessert (page 156).

4. PASTA

Pasta has received rave reviews as an excellent complex carbohydrate in the last 5 years. Perhaps obese Americans (10 lb. Pasta/year) are beginning to learn what much thinner Italians (70 lb. Pasta/year) have known for centuries. Pasta is a low fat, complex carbohydrate.

PASTA IS NUTRITIOUS, HEALTHY AND VERSATILE			
	CALORIES	PROTEIN	FAT UNITS
1 cup spaghetti or 1 1/2 cup macaroni	200	8 grams	1

The trick with pasta (like potatoes and bread and rice) is *not to ruin it* with *high fat* sauces and toppings. We include a number of excellent low fat pasta dishes in the recipe section. Most of the rice dishes are just as good on pasta. Try high protein pasta made from soy flour with a bit of garlic and a tablespoon of olive oil and a sprinkle of Parmesan cheese. Whole wheat pastas are excellent.

---

2 oz dry pasta =   1 cup spaghetti or noodles or 1½ cup macaroni

---

Beware of pre-packaged pastas with sauce (Sorry about the pasta-ronis, Billy!). Many are laced with salt and fat. Make spaghetti sauce in large batches and freeze meal size portions for fast and easy meals.

GEORGE'S BROCCOLI & GARLIC PASTA (Pg. 143)

1 1/2 Tbsp. Olive Oil
4 garlic cloves (finely chopped)
1 head (2 cups) broccoli (chopped)
4 cups of cooked spiral pasta
2 Tbsp. parmesan cheese

Cook pasta as above.
In large non-stick skillet, sauté garlic in olive oil. Add broccoli and cook until tender crisp.
Add cooked pasta and toss with parmesan cheese (and a squeeze of fresh lemon).
Serves 4
Calories - 200/serving
Fat Units - 7/serving

5. BEANS—THE MISUNDERSTOOD TREAT

Beans and peas and lentils are the most efficient source of vegetable protein. They are high in B vitamins and iron and low in fat. Beans provide all of the good things in meat with *no* harmful saturated *fats and the price is fantastic!*

FOOD	CALORIES	PROTEIN (grams)	FAT UNITS
LENTILS 8 oz (1 cup boiled)	231	18	1
LEAN BEEF 4 oz	360	32	24
KIDNEY BEANS 8 oz (1 cup)	225	15	1
BAKED BEANS CANNED 8 oz (1 cup)	250	11	4

See bean salad (pg. 117), lentil rice loaf (pg. 144), bean & corn salad (pg. 116), multi-bean soup (pg. 113) and lentil casserole (pg. 143) for great bean dishes. See the soup section for soups with lentils or mixed peas/beans. Obviously, the traditional hobo heating up baked beans in a tin knew how to eat well.

6. VEGGIES

Veggies are full of *fibre*, a storehouse of *vitamins* and *minerals*. They are *filling, crunchy* and *delicious*. Vegetables are great sources of the complex carbohydrates our bodies love. Remember to mix the types for a balance of vitamins and minerals. Deep yellow veggies such as carrots, pumpkin, squash and sweet potatoes contain valuable vitamin A. Deep green veggies such as spinach, chard and lettuce contain vitamins A and C, folic acid, iron and magnesium. Starchy veggies include corn, potatoes, green peas and sweet potatoes. These are excellent sources of low fat calories.

Try to have at least 2 vegetable servings a day–plus a big salad (with no-fat dressing) once a day. Eat until you are satisfied. God didn't make any bad veggies!

7. FRUIT—NATURE'S NECTAR

Enjoy at least 3 servings of fruit per day. They are low in calories, fat free and packed with vitamins (especially vitamin C). Eat your favorite fruits in abundance. Eat the fruit rather than drinking the juice (more fibre, more filling). Beware of sweetened juices.

FRUIT	CALORIES	FIBRE (grams)	FAT UNITS
Apple (medium)	80	3	0
Apple Juice (8 oz)	115	0	0

THE COMPLEX CARBOHYDRATES:

- *Fight and prevent heart disease*—by reducing obesity, high blood pressure and serum cholesterol.
- *Fight obesity*—by allowing steady weight loss with no hunger.
- *Fight diabetes*—by preventing sudden, harmful fluctuations in blood sugar in diabetics.
- *Fight the risk of cancer*—by eliminating the need for high fat foods (associated with breast cancer and bowel cancer) and by increasing fiber (reduces bowel cancer).

How about sugar—it's a carbohydrate—it must be good!

Sugar, in reasonable amounts is fine—(no fat units). *Pure sugars* such as white or brown granulated sugar or honey are *empty calories* (like alcohol). Pure sugars are high in calories without beneficial fibre, protein, vitamins or minerals.

* great complex carbohydrate   ** pure sugar

FOOD	CALORIES	FAT UNITS
** Coca Cola Classic (12 oz)	144	0
* 4 peaches	140	0
* 5 oz baked potato	160	0

The calories in a drink of coke could be replaced by 4 peaches plus a diet coke!

THE MESSAGE:

When it come to carbohydrates…be complex—not simple minded!

CARBOHYDRATE WARNING

You will notice that the high complex carbohydrate content of *"The Final Diet"* will give you a slight feeling of abdominal bloating *and*—shall we call it—flatulence (gas below!). These symptoms will only last a few weeks while your gut learns to make more enzymes (chemicals) to digest the great food you are eating. By the end of a month your gut will feel completely comfortable with this healthy diet.

Some people will experience a small weight gain (1–2 pounds) in the first week of the high carbohydrate, low fat final diet. We will explain that. The increase in carbohydrate will fill up the glycogen stores of the liver—stored 4 parts water to 1 part glycogen. Since the body holds 1 pound of glycogen (together with 4 pounds of water) there may be an initial small weight gain. The low fat content of *The Final Diet* will rapidly cause your body to burn *fat from fat cells* (held with very little water) and you will notice steady weight loss from the 2nd week on.

Don't despair if you have an initial small weight gain.

Your body will thrive on the Final Diet.
60% or more of your calories will come from the Super Seven.

THE SUPER SEVEN:
Grains (bread, cereals)
Potatoes
Rice
Pasta
Beans
Veggies
Fruit

CHAPTER 6

GREAT FOODS—PART 2:
TURKEY, CHICKEN (AND
FISH)—BIRDS OF PARADISE

You might think that calling a turkey or a chicken a bird of *paradise* is a bit far-fetched. However, we beg to differ. In fact, when passing poultry farms in the nearby countryside, we often get the urge to stop and give the big guys a cuddle (or let them give us a peck on the cheek!).

Animal protein is as good and useful to our body as vegetable protein. *Turkey, chicken and fish are wonderful sources of protein without the high fat that usually travels with animal protein.*

Meats, turkey, chicken, or fish should be barbecued, roasted broiled, microwaved or cooked in a non-stick pan or wok with minimal vegetable oil or cooking spray. Cooking by deep frying or cooking with butter or cream sauces adds huge numbers of Fat units to otherwise excellent food.

In the table on the following page, compare the calories, grams of protein and fat units per ounce of various meats and fishes. Turkey, chicken and fish are, indeed, birds of paradise.

ANIMAL PROTEIN SOURCES (ROASTED POULTRY, MEAT, FISH)

PROTEIN SOURCE	CALORIES/OZ.	GRAMS OF PROTEIN/OZ.	FAT UNITS/OZ.
* TURKEY BREAST W/O SKIN (1 oz)	40	8	1.5
* TURKEY DARK MEAT W/O SKIN (1 oz)	54	8	2
TURKEY LIGHT/DARK WITH SKIN (1 oz)	60	8	4
* CHICKEN BREAST W/O SKIN (1 oz)	50	8	1.5
* CHICKEN DARK W/O SKIN (1 oz)	60	8	3
CHICKEN DARK & LIGHT WITH SKIN (1 oz)	70	8	4
* HADDOCK, GROUPER, SOLE (1 oz) (ROASTED WITH BROTH/SPICES)	40	5	.5
GROUND LEAN BEEF (1 oz)	75	8	5
! LEAN LOIN BEEFSTEAK (1 oz)	80	8	5
! LEAN PORK TENDERLOIN (1 oz)	70	8	4
LEAN LAMB CHOP (1 oz)	70	8	4
BEEF SAUSAGE	90	4	8
PORK SAUSAGE	110	5	10

* LOW FAT PROTEIN SOURCES.

** lean cuts, roasted or broiled with fat removed.

The loin of beef or pork is a low fat cut.

In Canada, there are extra lean cuts of beef with as little as 3 fat units per oz (ask your butcher).

---

1 unit = 1 fat gram = 9 calories

Pig's tail takes the trophy as the most unattractive animal protein source—115 calories/ oz. With 10 fat units (90 calories of fat) per oz.!

Lean beef, pork and lamb are excellent sources of animal protein with higher fat content than poultry and fish.

TURKEY AND CHICKEN

Of the two birds of paradise, turkey has some advantages:
- cheaper (more meat per pound of carcass)
- easy to prepare and roast
- bigger (tons of leftovers–food for a week!)

TO ROAST TURKEY AND CHICKEN

Remove the skin—easy to do with a sharp knife and sharp scissors. You'll be amazed at the 4–5 lbs. of skin and fat that easily strip off a 20 lb. turkey. Sprinkle liberally with sage, thyme, black pepper and a pinch of garlic powder. Stuff with a delicious low-fat stuffing (pg. 126), cover with foil—and play tennis while supper (and food for a week) cooks.

FROZEN TURKEY AND CHICKEN BREASTS

These are wonderful to buy in bulk, free of skin and ready to marinate and barbecue or bake. You'll find many excellent recipes for turkey and chicken in chapter 16. Use these versatile birds for burgers, sandwiches, stews and lasagnas.

FISH-TURKEY OF THE SEA

Its hard to call fish a bird of paradise—but *fish is also packed with great protein with almost no fat.* Some fish have more fat than others:

FAT IN FISH

FISH	CALORIES/OZ.	FAT UNITS
LOW FAT Cod, Haddock, Lobster, Scallops, Bass, Perch, Pike, Shrimp	35	.5
CANNED TUNA PACKED IN WATER	36	.2
CRAB	30	.3
HIGHER IN FAT Trout, Salmon	50	2.5
Canned Tuna in oil	55	2

Fish oils have been shown to contain a fat (omega–3 fatty acid) that protects us from heart disease by lowering cholesterol and reducing blood clotting (the secret of Eskimos longevity in spite of eating whale blubber!). Therefore, even "high fat" fish is good for you.

Great protein wasted!

What we often do to these wonderful low fat proteins— turkey, chicken, fish—is roll them in batter (cod), dip them in butter (lobster) or cover them with bread crumbs and deep fry them (the colonel has no secrets!). The birds of paradise and the turkey of the sea die a miserable dietary death! Read the obituaries.

Obituaries

	CALORIES/OZ	FAT/GRAM	FAT CALORIES	FAT UNITS
"Light & Crispy" frozen fish fillets (battered & cooked in oil) - 1 oz.	90	5	45	5
Breaded & fried chicken nuggets - 1 oz.	75	5	45	5
Turkey patties, breaded & fried - 1 oz.	90	5	45	5

Great protein becomes high fat, high calorie food!

The problem:

1 tbsp. Vegetable oil = 120 calories (all vegetable fat)
1 tbsp. Butter = 110 calories (all animal fat)
1 tbsp. Margarine = 100 calories (all vegetable fat)

These excellent foods must be baked, barbecued or roasted with low fat sauces to maintain their food value! We'll teach you more about that in the next few chapters and provide great low fat recipes.

A FEW LAST THOUGHTS ABOUT GREAT PROTEIN:

•   Your daily protein need is about 70 grams (.4 grams/lb.). For a 160 lb. person. Most meats/poultry/fish have 5–7 grams per oz. A good diet might fill that protein/ oz. requirement as follows:

FOOD & PORTION	GRAMS OF PROTEIN
8 oz. skim milk (needed for calcium)	8
6 oz. (3/4) cup no-fat yogurt	8
6 oz. meat/turkey/chicken/fish	36
4 pieces of bread per day	10
8 oz (1 cup) pasta/potatoes/rice	5
veggies/fruit	5
TOTAL	72

NOTE:
  *   Beans (lentils, baked beans, kidney, lima, etc.) are wonderful sources of protein (also low in fat).
  *   All portions can be expanded or shrunk for those ideal weights higher or lower than 160 lbs.

•   With high protein/low fat meat, poultry and fish—more than 4 oz. can be eaten without exceeding total daily fat unit and calorie goals.

Chapter 7

Great Foods—Part 3:
Low Fat Dairy Products—Healthy Protein

The slim six

- Skim milk
- No-fat yogurt
- 1% cottage cheese
- skim milk
- frozen yogurt
- frozen sherbet (sorbet)
- 1% ice cream

Dairy products are an excellent source of several nutrients essential to human health:

- **Protein:**

The slim six provide good animal protein with little or no harmful animal (saturated) fat.

- **Calcium:**

We need 800 mg. of calcium per day (2 x 8 oz glasses of skim milk or2 cups of non-fat yogurt) to provide for good solid bone structure and other important body functions.

COMMON DAIRY PRODUCTS
WITH CALORIES, PROTEIN AND FAT UNITS

DAIRY PRODUCT	CALORIES	PROTEIN (gm)	FAT UNITS
MILK			
* SKIM MILK (8oz)	90	8.5	0
1% milk (8oz)	100	8	3
2% milk (8oz)	120	8	5
3.5% (whole) milk (8oz)	150	8	8
YOGURT * NO FAT YOGURT (4oz) Plain or fruit	56	6	0
Low fat yogurt (4oz) - fruit	110	4.5	1.5
Regular plain yogurt	125	4.5	2.5

DAIRY PRODUCTS TABLE-CONTINUED...

DAIRY PRODUCT	CALORIES	PROTEIN	FAT UNITS
CHEESE			
*1% COTTAGE CHEESE (4oz = ½ cup)	80	14	2
Creamed Cottage Cheese (4oz)	120	14	5
Skim milk cheese (2oz)	160	12	12
Cheddar, Colby, Process Cheese (2oz)	225	14	16
1% Ultra Light cheese slices (.6oz)	30	4.6	.2
* SKIM MILK FROZEN YOGURT (3.5oz)	110	2	2
* FROZEN SHERBET (3.5oz) (Sorbet)	110	1	1
Ice Cream (3.5oz)	240	5	15
* 1% ICE CREAM (3.5oz)	105	3	1

The slim six

Skim milk

2 glasses of skim milk a day are an excellent way to provide 17 grams of protein (of 70 grams needed per day) plus the entire day's calcium supply. If you presently drink 2% milk switch to skim milk using the following schedule:

Week 1–mix 2% and 1% milk half and half
Week 2–drink 1% milk
Week 3–mix 1% and skim milk half and half
Week 4–drink skim milk (ice cold–it's great!)

No fat yogurt

Take a cup of plain no-fat yogurt (112 calories) and add ⅔ cup of fresh fruit (peaches, grapes, bananas, black currents, raspberries….). Add ½ tsp. of sweetener (brown sugar Twin is good) and ½ tsp. vanilla extract. Mix and eat! No fat yogurt makes a great breakfast (with a low fat muffin, recipe pg. 97-99 or a crunchy piece of whole wheat toast and jam)–a great lunch (with a whole wheat raisin bun, recipe page 95) or a super dessert for under 150 calories (0 fat).

New! No fat yogurt with fruit—only 55 calories and no fat per 4 oz serving.

No fat yogurt, low calories with no fat, has an excellent taste and can be used for a topping on fruit or as a garnish on baked potatoes.

1% cottage cheese

Mix this low-fat, high protein food with blueberries, melon or pineapple and we have a filling lunch (with a bagel). Put it in lasagna in place of high fat cheese. It is great with chives and onions on baked potatoes in place of sour cream. 1% cottage cheese is delicious, nutritious and almost fat-free.

Frozen (skim milk) yogurt–too good to be true

We can't believe that a product as delicious as black cherry frozen yogurt could be good for you! (110 calories and 2 fat units per 3.5 oz). This food is a perfect dessert.

FROZEN SHERBET (SORBET)

Delicious and versatile, sherbet has a lighter taste than ice cream or frozen yogurt and is great with fruit. It has 110 calories with 1 fat unit per 3.5 oz serving.

1% ICE CREAM

Try butterscotch or chocolate cherry mint 1% ice cream at 105 calories per 3.5 oz serving with less than 1 fat unit. It is incredibly delicious. It should be fattening, but it's not; it's excellent food.

A new low fat dairy product!
1% Ultra Light Process Cheese slices
30 calories and .2 fat units per slice.
Great for sandwiches.

ON THE HORIZON:

No fat Philadelphia cream cheese by Kraft at 25 calories/ oz (no fat) is available in the U.S.A. but not in Canada. No fat cottage cheese will be available in the next year in North America. The food industry is very creative.

1% sour cream is now available in Canada and the U.S.A. with only 26 calories and .4 fat units per 2 tablespoons. It is excellent for baked potatoes.

CHAPTER 8

THE FAT TRAPS—HOW TO BEAT THEM

We now expose the *common fat traps*–the reason why 30% of North Americans are overweight and suffering from nutritional (over nutrition?) diseases.

FAT TRAP #1:

JUNK FOOD-SNACKS, SWEETS, GOODIES

These foods appeared in North America in the 1950s and 1960s. Consumption has reached epidemic proportions! They are the #1 cause of obesity in our society. *Although we blame sugar, the culprit is truly fat,* making up 80% of the calories in these foods.

BAD SNACKS

In this list we will recognize many of our favorite treats. The fat content is shocking.

See table on page following.

FOOD	CALORIES	FAT UNITS	% OF TOTAL CALORIES AS FAT CALORIES
Chocolate Bars (average size)	300	20	60%
Ice Cream Bar	250	15	54%
Potato Chips (40-small bag)	400	26	59%
Nachos (2 cups)	360	12	30%
Chocolate Chip Cookies (2 medium)	110	5	41%
Cheese Crackers (10)	100	6.5	59%
Butter Popcorn (3 cups)	190	10	47%
Chocolate Coated Almonds (6)	161	12	67%
Peanuts (1oz - 50 nuts)	160	14	79%
Cashews (1oz - 16 nuts)	160	13	73%

1 fat unit = 1 gram of fat = 9 calories

Fat trap #1: snacks–the solution

- Avoid excessive hunger caused by skipping breakfast and/or lunch. Pack wholesome bag lunches with filling, healthy food. Avoid snack attacks–especially if your work or leisure puts you in irregular schedules or stressful situations with easy access to junk food.

- Eat wholesome 'snack food' as soon as you feel hungry. Carry fresh fruit when you travel—in a small cooler! You will notice that "The Final Diet" fills you up at meal times and that you feel pleasant hunger again 3–4 hours after meals–just before the next meal.

- If you need something *sweet*, try lifesavers—(10 calories each); *or* a bottle of diet pop—(1 calorie) to satisfy your craving.

GREAT SNACK FOOD

Here are some excellent healthy treats.

FOOD	CALORIES	FAT UNITS
Medium apple, orange, 2 plums or 2 peaches (or 1 serving of most fruits)	80	0
Raw veggies (2 cups) with no-fat yogurt dip (Recipe page 105)	60	0
3 cups air popped popcorn	80	0
20 pretzels (1 oz)	110	1
1 piece whole wheat raisin toast with (1 Tbsp.) light jam (double fruit, half the sugar jam!)	120 30	1 0
4 oz. delicious frozen yogurt or sherbet or 1% ice cream	110	3

FAT TRAP #2: FAST FOOD

Fast food, including many prepared frozen meals, is the #2 cause of obesity in north America. Again these foods appeared in the 1950s and 1960s when the population got cars (to visit the golden arches) and freezers (to freeze those pot pies and pizzas). The calorie content and fat units in most fast foods is absolutely revolting! See the fast food section of the food list (chapter 17).

Here are the disturbing calorie and fat unit contents of North America's favorites.

FOOD	CALORIES	FAT UNITS
Deep Fried Chicken - 2 pieces (6oz)	470	27
Fish Sandwich (deep fried with cheese)	421	23
Onion Rings - small serving (3oz)	285	16
French Fries - small	227	13
Double Cheeseburger with bacon	510	31
Chocolate Shake	320	12
Caramel Sundae	360	10
Cherry Pie (snack pie)	357	13
Carrot Muffin	260	14

FAT TRAP #2: FAST FOODS-THE SOLUTION

- *Avoid all fast food restaurants!*
  When you travel or need a quick meal on the road–
  pack a lunch. Eat deep fried food regularly and you
  will become obese! *The best 'quick' food is a
  Turkey sub sandwich*—no mayo, no butter, no
  cheese, whole wheat bun, lots of lettuce, mustard,
  onions, and peppers. It tastes great and is low in fat!

- *When buying frozen or microwave dinners,* buy only
  those with a label of calories, fat and contents. Some
  are excellent–some are terrible! Most of the entrée
  recipes in this book require less than 15 minutes to
  prepare—especially the pasta and rice with stir-fry
  toppings. We recommend that you save money and
  needless calories by cooking home-made meals.

- If you don't know where your next meal is coming
  from—*pack a lunch.*

FAT TRAP #3: GOOD BREAD/BAD SPREADS

Butter, margarine and peanut butter spell trouble for the fat
budget! This following table illustrates the problem with high fat
spreads.
"Bad" spreads can turn wonderful fresh bread (70 calories/
½" slice) into a high fat, high calorie food!! At 9 calories per fat

FOOD	CALORIES	FAT UNITS
Butter - 1 tbsp.	108	12
Light Butter - 1 tbsp.	54	6
Margarine (safflower) - 1 tbsp.	102	12
Diet Margarine - 1 tbsp.	51	6
Peanut Butter - 1 tbsp.	95	8

unit, all of the calories in butter and margarine and 70% of the calories in peanut butter *come from fat.*

FAT TRAP #3: SPREADS-THE SOLUTION

- If you really enjoy a high fat spread on bread–switch to diet margarine–half the calories and half the fat (vegetable fat). Use safflower or sunflower margarine.

- Make your own bread (recipe page 95) *or* find an excellent bakery to buy fresh whole wheat bread. Heat it in the microwave (10 seconds/slice) or toast it. Cover it *thickly* with 1 tbs. Of *ultra light fruit jam* (20 calories/tbs.—No fat). This excellent jam (raspberry, strawberry, mixed fruit, blueberry) is available in supermarkets. There is *more fruit* and *less added sugar.* We stopped using any butter or margarine at our house—we all love the delicious flavor of fresh bread or toast with fruit. (ultra light double fruit jam is made in Canada by culinary and by president's choice and is available in the U.S.A.)

- Switch from peanut butter to jam.

- Don't put butter or margarine or sour cream on baked or mashed potatoes. Use 1% cottage cheese or no-fat yogurt mixed with chives or green onions. Save 80 calories and 9 fat units each time you have a baked potato! (1 tsp. butter/2 tbs. sour cream). 1% sour cream is also fine (26 calories and .4 fat units/2 tbs.)

- Use spices–parsley, pepper, garlic powder, coriander, basil, thyme, cinnamon or curry powder on vegetables. Forget the high fat butter and margarine.

FAT TRAP #4: MAYONNAISE

Excellent foods such as potatoes (salad) and turkey (sandwich) become "mine-fields" of fat by adding mayonnaise. *Salad bars are the greatest low-cal hoax on the planet.* In salad bars, cups of mayonnaise and gallons of fat units are hidden in the pasta salads, potato salads, coleslaws and dressings attractively displayed with healthy vegetables and leafs of lettuce. A healthy Caesar salad may have several hundred calories of fat in a mayonnaise based dressing.

MAYONNAISE:

From wicked to righteous: no fat mayonnaise has arrived!

FOOD	CALORIES	FAT UNITS
REGULAR MAYONNAISE 1 tbsp.	100	11
LIGHT MAYONNAISE 1 tbsp.	50	5.5
<u>*NO FAT* MAYONNAISE</u> 1 tbsp.	12	0

FAT TRAP #4: MAYONNAISE-THE SOLUTION

- No fat mayonnaise–looks, tastes and behaves exactly like real mayonnaise; but it has 12 calories/tbs. And no fat!

We can enjoy those foods that normally *need* mayonnaise–potato salad (recipes pages 151–153), turkey, lettuce and tomato sandwich (recipe page 100), creamy Caesar salad dressing (recipe page 118), pasta salads (recipe page 122) and scrumptious coleslaw (recipe page 119). This product is made in Canada by president's choice and in the U.S.A. By Kraft. This wonderful new food is *not* made from nuclear waste–it's natural vegetable products.

FAT TRAP #5: SALAD DRESSINGS

Salad is a wonderful healthy food. A huge bowl (3 cups) of mixed lettuce, onions, peppers, carrots, celery and tomatoes is less than 50 calories (no fat). However, everyone puts at least 2 tbs. Of salad dressing on salads. Chosen poorly, salad dressings can easily bankrupt both calorie goals and fat unit budgets!

SALAD DRESSINGS:

This table illustrates the benefits of new, low fat dressings.

FOOD	CALORIES	FAT UNITS
REGULAR DRESSING		
French 2 tbsp.	134	13
Italian 2 tbsp.	140	14
LOW CALORIE DRESSING		
French 2 tbsp.	44	2
Italian 2 tbsp.	32	3
NO FAT DRESSING		
French 2 tbsp.	30	.5
Italian 2 tbsp.	10	0
NO FAT HOMEMADE CAESAR (Pg.118)	15	0

FAT TRAP #5: SALAD DRESSINGS-THE SOLUTION

- Enjoy huge bowls of salad with 2–3 tbs. Of *no fat dressing*. Dine until you are full with a clear conscience! These are excellent foods.

FAT TRAP #6: DESSERTS

Desserts are a trap for those of us with a sweet tooth (often a fat tooth!) Bad desserts are high in simple sugars but also high in fat units.

BAD DESSERTS

Most of us have intimate relations with these culprits.

FOOD	CALORIES	FAT UNITS
Frozen Apple Spice Cake (4oz - medium piece)	420	18
Double Fudge Brownies (2") (2 - no one eats one!)	360	12
Cherry Cheese Cake - small piece	400 (at least!)	24
Ice Cream (4oz)	250	16

FAT TRAP #6: DESSERTS-THE SOLUTION

Low calorie desserts are possible *and* as delicious as high calories/high fat desserts. Desserts provide a sweet and light taste at the end of a meal, when we are satisfied from good protein and complex carbohydrates.

EXCELLENT DESSERTS

Here are a few listed with calories and fat units.

FOOD	CALORIES	FAT UNITS
4 oz Black Cherry Frozen Yogurt	110	3
1 cup mixed fresh fruit with no fat yogurt topping	100	0
1 cup cold green grapes plus a peach	110	0

We suggest you limit desserts to 150 calories and 3 fat units. We include a list of *21 super desserts under 150 calories* in the *dessert recipes* (page 158).

FAT TRAP #7

HIGH CALORIE OR HIGH FAT DRINKS

Many drinks create a food trap because of their high content of calories (not fat). In the case of whole (3.7%) milk or cream– a fat trap can also be present.

DRINKS (HIGH CALORIE)

It is amazingly easy to take a large portion of our daily calorie in liquid form.

FOOD	CALORIES	FAT UNITS
Orange Juice - frozen (8oz)	120	0
Apple Juice (8oz)	120	0
Lemonade - frozen (8oz)	130	0
Beer - regular (12oz)	150	0
Table Wine (4oz)	80	0
Regular Pop (12oz)	150	0
Whole Milk 3.7% (8oz)	157	9
Table Cream (1oz)	60	6

FAT TRAP #7: HIGH CALORIE OR HIGH FAT DRINKS–THE SOLUTION

EXCELLENT DRINKS:

These are the drinks that quench thirst without excessive calories or fat.

FOOD	CALORIES	FAT UNITS
Ice water (6-8 8oz glasses/day)	0	0
Coffee/tea (8oz)	2-5	0
Skim milk (8oz)	87	0
Diet pop (12oz)	1-4	0
Light Beer (12oz)	100	0

It is helpful to get calories from food rather than from beverages.

- *Instead of fruit juices–eat the apple or orange & 1 glass of ice water.*
  In doing so, we get *all* of the nutrients, vitamins and all of the fibre in the fruit. Also, the filling effect of fibre plus water reduces food intake and promotes weight loss.

- *Drink 6–8 large glasses of ice water daily–water is the only fluid our bodies require.*
  Keep ice water or carbonated water (expensive) in the refrigerator at all times. Slices of lime or lemon and loose ice cubes (in the freezer) make water more interesting and appetizing. Consider purchasing a fridge with an ice cube maker on the door. They quickly repay the extra expense by making nature's beverage, water, more attractive and available.

- *Coffee/tea*
  With milk or cream and sugar, coffee and tea can contain up to 80 calories and 4 fat units per cup. Many obese people trace their problem to 6–8 cups of coffee with cream and sugar per day. We suggest you switch to "black" tea and coffee. Taken "black", your intake of these drinks will drop (100 milligrams of caffeine per brewed cup of coffee!). As you rediscover the true taste of tea and coffee your interest in them will return and you'll have a chance to set a limit of 2–3 cups per day.

SWEETENERS

ASPARTAME

(Nutri-sweet) aspartame has become one of the hottest food items in the world in the last few years. (The sweetener in diet coke or diet Pepsi). It has had more scientific testing and scrutiny than any other food on the planet. Except for rare cases of headache and several "possible" cases of seizure related to this sweetener, it has been shown to have *no* harmful effects.

Health and welfare Canada suggest a limit (18 mg./lb) in the consumption of aspartame which totals 14 cans (10 oz) of diet pop per day for a 150 lb. Person. It would appear that our bladders would fail before we could harm ourselves with this product. Sweeteners have no effect on food intake or appetite. These products can be used in moderation (3–4 cans of pop/day) if you enjoy sweet tasting calorie free drinks. The diet colas contain half the caffeine of brewed coffee (50 mg. vs. 100 mg. for 8 oz).

Artificial sweeteners are useful in modest amounts. They add sweetness to foods with no known health risk.

Saccharin brown sugar substitute

This is a useful substitute (tsp. For tsp.) For brown sugar in dessert recipes. At 1 calories/tsp. It has 1/10 of the calories of brown sugar (20 calories/tsp.). It is *excellent* for sweetening fruit, yogurt or vegetables (e.g. Super squash pg. 120) but performs poorly when baked with flour.

Splenda (the new sweetener)

This sweetener has recently been approved for use in both the U.S.A. And Canada. Being new, it's cumulative effects on humans are not well understood. We would suggest caution in using more than small amounts until it has been on the market for a few more years. Splenda appears to be a useful product for baking.

CHAPTER 9

A REVIEW—SMART SUBSTITUTIONS

THE PROBLEM	THE SMART (LOW-FAT) SUBSTITUTE
SNACKS chocolate bars, potato chips, ice cream, butter popcorn	fruit, low-fat frozen yogurt, no-fat yogurt with fruit, frozen sorbet, 1% ice cream, air popped popcorn, pretzels
crackers, cookies	bread with fruit jam, Wasa Crisps, saltine crackers with jam
FAST FOOD burgers	Turkey sub with no cheese, no mayonnaise, (lots of onions, lettuce, mustard). Pack a lunch.
fries	rice, pasta (without cream sauces), baked potatoes
donuts, high fat muffins	bread, rolls, bagel or toast with jam
prepacked frozen dinners	simple home-made dinners (see chapter 15) for 2 weeks of great, fast, home cooked low fat suppers.
SPREADS butter, margarine, peanut butter	low cal fruit jams, honey (in moderation) or eat fresh bread plain (it's great!).
MAYONNAISE All fat (100 calories/Tbsp.)	**NO FAT MAYONNAISE** - No Fat! (12 calories/Tbsp.)
SALAD DRESSINGS Regular dressings are all fat (135 calories/2 Tbsp.)	**NO FAT SALAD DRESSING** - (30 calories/2 Tbsp.) No fat caesar dressing (page 118). * Take no fat salad dressing along when you eat in a restaurant.
DESSERTS Cakes, Pies, etc.	**LOW FAT/LOW CALORIE** - see page 158 of Recipe section for 21 great low fat desserts. *All under* 150 calories!!

Smart substitutions table–cont'd.

THE PROBLEM	THE SMART (LOW-FAT) SUBSTITUTE
HIGH CALORIE DRINKS . *juices*	**GOOD DRINKS** *eat the fruit (filling, fibre) plus water*
pop	*diet pop (in moderation), <u>ice water</u> (the best by far!)*
alcohol	*light alcohol, diet drinks, mineral water, dilute drinks with ice or water*
high fat dairy drinks (cream, milk)	*skim milk (no fat)*
HIGH FAT PROTEIN *fatty beef, pork, lamb, poultry skin*	**LOW FAT PROTEIN** *turkey, chicken, fish, seafood, ultra lean beef, ultra lean pork*
whole eggs (80 cal., 6 fat units)	*egg white (11 cal., NO FAT)*
HIGH FAT DAIRY PRODUCTS	**LOW FAT DAIRY PRODUCTS**
milk, cheese, ice cream	*skim milk, 1% cottage cheese, frozen yogurt, frozen sherbet and 1% ice cream*

OBESITY PREVENTION RULES

- Know what is in it before you put it in your mouth! (We all treat our pets that well).

- If there is no nutrient information (calories/protein/ fat per serving) on the package *-don't buy it!* The food producer may not be entirely proud of the contents of the food.

- If it's bad stuff and you feel hungry—eat something good.

- If you are visiting and don't want to offend your host (offering you black forest cake), say you just ate or say you are cutting back on desserts (but it looks wonderful).

- Eat lots of super seven complex carbohydrates (grain products—bread & cereals, potatoes, rice, pasta, beans, veggies, fruit).

CHAPTER 10

SURVIVAL KIT FOR DINING OUT

• *Avoid restaurants that serve nothing but fast food.* (i.e. burgers, fries, onion rings, milk shakes, etc.). They will surely try to pack an ounce or two of fat back on our increasingly slim bodies!

• GOOD, SAFE RESTAURANT FOODS

Salads: mixed green, seafood, are great *if* there is a reduced calorie dressing available. Ask for dressing as a side order. Better yet, take along your own no-fat salad dressing and eat all the salad and dressing you want. Beware of pre-mixed Caesar salads, potato salads and pasta salads at salad bars (mayonnaise).

Fresh bread & rolls: these are great. Ask for jam instead of butter—if they serve breakfast, they will have jam.

Soups: usually home-made soups are broth-based, and delicious. Opt for vegetable or barley soups. Avoid creamed soups which often contain cream or high fat thickener.

Meat: Grilled meat, poultry or fish is the best. Avoid deep fried food (e.g. shrimp). Watch out for high calorie toppings on meat–ask the server what the sauces contain and ask for them on entrees.

Sandwiches: sandwiches are excellent foods in restaurants. Ask for a turkey or chicken breast sub or sandwich–hold the mayonnaise and butter. Add lots of tomato, onion, pickles, mustard, pepper—delicious and safe.

Veggies: without butter, cheese sauce or other high fat topping, vegetables are tasty and low in fat and calories.

Baked potatoes/rice/pasta: these are super foods. Don't ruin them with sour cream or butter!

Pasta: assume that meat sauce will not be made from lean meat. Ask for a half order of meat sauce with a full order of pasta. This is a good way to assess the tip that you plan for the server (Attitude assessment!).

Desserts: skip them! They are expensive and usually arrive loaded with fat and sugar. Pop into the grocery store on the way home and buy black cherry frozen yogurt and enjoy a low fat, low calorie treat at a fraction of the price. Many good restaurants will have sherbet or frozen yogurt on the menu.

Eating in restaurants is a necessary way of life for many people. Learn to travel with a small ice chest that contains a survival kit–skim milk, high fibre cereal, fruit, no-fat yogurt or cottage cheese, fresh bread and jam. Remember to *pack a lunch* when you know that you will find yourself hungry in a setting where only high fat, high calorie foods will be available.

With some thought and foresight, we can leave home without threatening dietary disaster.

Chapter 11

Exercise—the Second Essential

A slim, fit, healthy body is the result of diet plus exercise. Exercise alone will not overcome a high calorie, fat laden diet. Diet alone will not overcome an inactive, sedentary life-style.

To shed a pound of fat we must use up
3500 calories of energy that we don't eat.

Cutting Calories
- Eat enough to support our ideal weight (not our "over weight").
- Burn off calories exercising at least 4 times per week.

We treat our bodies like the lean, fit, machines that they *will* become.

There Are Excellent Scientific Reasons to Exercise:

1. Exercise prevents muscle loss as we reduce our food intake to promote weight loss. With no exercise—our weight loss is partly muscle. Muscle is *the most* active energy burner in the body. Therefore, we reduce our

body's total daily energy *needs* if we lose muscle. We put weight back on with *less* food intake than before weight loss. This process of muscle loss, plus water loss and gain, is the *yo-yo effect* common with starvation diet programs under 1200 calories per day.

2. Exercise reduces anxiety and depression and promotes a feeling of well being!   A happy hormone called endorphin is released–a cheap and healthy high.

3. Regular exercise is vital to maintain a healthy heart and blood circulatory system.   It builds stronger bone, reduces blood pressure and heart rate and protects against the effects of cholesterol.

4. *Exercise burns fat from our fat cells and makes us lean.*

Table 11a lists calories burned per hour for popular forms of work and exercise for a 150 pound person.

TABLE 11A

| CALORIES BURNED PER 60 MINUTES OF EXERCISE ||
EXERCISE	CALORIES/60 MIN.
WORK:	
Digging, moving lumber	600
Mowing grass (pushing power mower)	400
Painting house	300
Scrubbing floor	400
Sweeping, vacuuming	200
SPORTS:	
Badminton	300
Bowling	200
Cross-Country Skiing (brisk)	800
Cross-Country Skiing (lazy)	400
Cycling (brisk)	600
Cycling (lazy)	400
Down Hill Skiing	400
Skipping Rope	600
Squash/Raquetball/Handball	600
Swimming (brisk)	400
Tennis	400
Walking (brisk)	400
Water Skiing	400
RUNNING:	
12 minute miles	600
8 minute miles	800
6 minute miles	1000
Stepping Machines	300-800
Stationary Bicycles	400-600

[handwritten in margin: 660-M / 540-A]

These figures are for a 150 pound man or woman. For each 15 pounds over 150 pounds, add 10% to calories/hour. For each 15 pounds under 150 pounds, subtract ·10% from calories/hour. e.g. If a 180 pound man walks briskly for 1 hour, he burns a total of 400 + (20% of 400) = 480 calories.

HOW TO EXERCISE TO MAKE THE FAT REVOLUTION
WORK FOR YOU.

- Pick an exercise you enjoy. If you hate all exercise pick brisk walking.

- Buy a wrist watch with a stop watch (available under $15.00) to time your exercise and your pulse.

- Dress comfortably with good footwear and sweat socks.

- If you are over 40 and out of shape, please don't take up running! (We don't need honorable mention in anyone's obituary!) If you are over 40 and really want to do aggressive exercise–see your physician for a stress EKG and physical exam. If you have any health problems or concerns see your doctor to discuss the best exercise.

- *Schedule exercise into your day's routine* like meals and banking and haircuts. It is important.

- If you enjoy companionship schedule exercise with a friend (e.g. racquetball 3 times/week). If you enjoy solitude and a chance to clear your mind (a lot of us with people jobs or big families need it!)–use your exercise period as a sanity break. We love to tune out from the world with lovely music (via Walkman) while cross-country skiing, using a stepping machine or using a stationary bike.

- If you haven't been exercising, start with brisk walking for 20 minutes. Build up the time and the intensity of your exercise. A gradual increase encourages persistence and reduces achy muscles.

- Do 45 minutes of your favorite exercise at least 4 times a week. From table 11a, if you exercise 5 days/week, you use from 750 calories/week bowling to 3000 calories/week cross-country skiing (if you weigh 150 pounds).

THE BEST EXERCISE-AEROBIC

Aerobic exercise is best for heart/lung/muscle training *and* for burning calories. The goal of *aerobic* exercise is to work our bodies hard enough to increase our heart rate to 60 to 80% of maximum for over 30 minutes. Aerobic exercise is *any physical* activity that produces that change in our heart rate.

Note: check your pulse now at your carotid artery (on the side of your neck about 2" outside the middle of your throat). Count your pulse for 15 seconds and multiply by 4. You can do this while exercising to maintain your pulse in the aerobic range. Table 11b, below, shows us aerobic ranges (60 to 80% of maximum) according to age.

TABLE 11B: AEROBIC HEART RATE RANGE FOR AGE

During aerobic exercise, the body burns energy (including stored fat) very efficiently. For our bodies, exercise is like getting a locomotive out of the shed to use the engines efficiently. *Aerobic exercise produces weight loss (especially fat!) and fitness, when combined with a rational healthy diet.*

Exercise experts know that our metabolism stays "sped up"

AGE	AEROBIC HEART RATE RANGE/MINUTE
20	120 - 160
25	115 - 155
30	115 - 150
35	110 - 150
40	110 - 140
45	105 - 140
50	100 - 135
55	100 - 130
60	95 - 130
65+	95 - 120

for several hours after exercise, thus burning more calories. Sustained (30 min.) aerobic exercise is the best exercise for burning fat. The best time to exercise is before meals.

Some people fail at exercise programs because they attempt difficult competitive sports requiring athletic ability (e.g. squash). Many people take a trial (3 month) membership at a fitness club to find a suitable exercise activity. When you find *your* exercise, it becomes a favorite part of your day. Biking (aerobic), cross-country skiing (aerobic), tennis (fun), combined with weight training (for muscle strength) are our favorite ways to burn calories and keep fit. Brisk walking is an inexpensive and enjoyable exercise easily available to everyone.

Start today–exercise at least 4 times per week for 45 minutes–you'll quickly get to love it!

ANAEROBIC EXERCISE

Short intense exercise (e.g. 10 minutes of hard running) quickly exhausts the body's oxygen capacity and is called *an*aerobic (no oxygen) exercise. Noxious chemicals, especially lactic acid, are produced that makes us feel achy, drained and sometimes nauseated. Anaerobic exercise is not recommended in this book unless you enjoy aggressive competition.

EXERCISE: A REVIEW

- *Exercise is necessary, with The Final Diet, to achieve a healthy lean body.*
- Brisk exercise (45 minutes four times/week) will ensure that the great majority of body weight lost on the Final Diet will be body fat, not muscle.
- Aerobic exercise (heart rate 60 to 80% of maximum) is the best exercise for fitness and fat burning!
- Schedule exercise into your day's activities.

A FINAL THOUGHT ON EXERCISE:

To actually *improve* your physique while on *"The Final Diet/*

exercise program" combine aerobic activity (45 minutes three times a week) with a muscle building activity (45 minutes two times a week). Muscle building activities include heavy outside work (digging, chopping wood), swimming, rowing, home exercises, weight lifting, (nautilus circuits or free weights) and many fitness group classes (dance-aerobics with small weights).

"The only reason I would take up jogging, is to hear heavy breathing again."
E. Bombeck

Chapter 12

Cholesterol—A Few Words of Advice

Adults should see their doctors to arrange for a blood test to measure fasting levels of cholesterol (and other fats). Young people (age 10–18) with a family history of heart attacks under age 60 should have the same blood tests.

Research has shown that foods high in saturated fat (animal fat) are the main cause of raised blood cholesterol. If our cholesterol level is high or high normal, we should:

- Achieve ideal weight–in over 80% of people, cholesterol will return to normal.
- Follow a low fat, high complex carbohydrate diet such as *The Final Diet*.
- Avoid high cholesterol foods as much as possible.
- Follow a regular aerobic exercise program.
- Have repeat blood cholesterol tests after 6 months.
- If levels remain high, there are excellent cholesterol lowering drugs.

Each 1% drop in blood cholesterol reduces the risk of death by heart disease by 2%.

HIGH CHOLESTEROL FOODS

High cholesterol foods include egg yolks, butter, shrimp and fatty meats. Lean meats, poultry, fish, skim milk, no fat dairy products are low in cholesterol. The body makes cholesterol as a result of saturated fat in the diet.

CAN I EAT EGGS?

Egg whites are great. All of the fat *and* cholesterol in an egg is in the yolk! A large egg has 80 calories and 6 fat units. The white has 11 calories and no fat or cholesterol! Egg yolk should be limited to 2 to 4 per week if you have normal cholesterol! For a delicious low cholesterol, low fat omelet, see recipe on page 101.

CHAPTER 13

THE FINAL DIET—LET'S GO!!

THE FINAL DIET IN REVIEW:

- My *calorie goal* is_____ (count for 2 weeks)
  My *fat unit goal* is_____ (count for 4 weeks)

- Chapter 15 contains meal plans for 2 weeks to get started.

- Now we have the knowledge to fight fat.

THE PRINCIPLES:

- *Excess fat in food is the main cause of obesity and the related diseases.*
- *Reduce daily fat intake to 15 to 20% (or less) of calories to reach daily fat goal.*
- *Eat adequate protein daily (70 grams)..*
- *Use the super seven complex carbohydrates to provide over 60% of daily calories.*
- *Eat 3 satisfying meals per day (no hunger).!*
- *Exercise 45 minutes or more at least 4 times per week.*

Chapter 14

Common Questions

Question #1

My calorie goal is 1500 calories/day on *"The Final Diet."* Can I drop my calories to 1000/day and cut my fat units drastically to lose weight faster?

Answer #1

Do not cut your calories under 1200 calories/day or you will experience all the symptoms of starvation. Also, you will probably quit *"The Final Diet"* and yo-yo back up to your original weight (or more).

You can safely cut your fat units to 17 fat units (which is 10% of total calories). However, if you do, you should ensure that this fat is in the form of good vegetable oil to satisfy your body's essential fat needs. Probably the best approach is to take 15% of calories as fat as your goal, if you are in a rush. Increasing exercise up to 1 hour or more 5 times per week would also accelerate weight loss!

Our suggestion is to be patient. Obesity is a problem that takes years to develop and should be approached gently. *"The Final Diet"* will help you make good food choices that will help you eat intelligently–for life. Over weeks (or months) you will lose weight and regain your fitness.

Therefore, the best advice we can give is to follow the 15%

fat unit goal and get lots of exercise. And think of long term success.

QUESTION #2

I love potatoes and whole wheat raisin bread. They are complex carbohydrates–so, I can eat all I want! Right?

ANSWER #2

Not exactly! Both potatoes and bread are excellent carbohydrates that supply fibre, minerals and vitamins with little fat.

However, if you have 15 pieces of raisin bread per day (70 x 15 = 1050 calories) it would use up the bulk of your days calories. You certainly could tolerate 4–5 pieces of bread and 2 baked potatoes per day if you enjoy them.

The next chapter contains 2 weeks of sample menus to help you focus on a healthy mix of complex carbohydrates (65%) with protein (15%) and fat (15–20%).

QUESTION #3

I am a 5'10" man, medium build, who weighs 200 pounds. How fast will I lose weight *on The Final Diet*? I plan to continue playing vigorous racquetball 4 days/week at lunch time.

ANSWER #3

At 5'10" your ideal weight is 165 pounds (table 4a) and your calorie goal is 2150 calories/day. Your fat unit goal is 36–48 fat units/day (15–20% range) (table 4c).

Your 200 pound body *thinks* it wants 3800 calories/day (19 calories/pound). You will give it 2150 calories/day (or less) by eating more complex carbohydrates and cutting fat.

Food savings (3800–2150) x 7 days = 11,550 calories/week.

Your vigorous racquetball (600 calories/hour) will be very helpful for burning calories. Since you weigh 200 pounds your body will burn more than the 600 calories/hour that a 150 pound person would per hour of racquetball. For each 15 pounds over

150 pounds you will use an extra 10% of calories. Therefore you will burn 130% of 600 calories per hour or 780 calories per hour. This projects to approximately 600 calories per 45 minute game.

Exercise savings = 600 calories/game x 4 days/week = 2400 calories
Total calories saved = 13,950 per week

Since 3500 = 1 pound loss, you will lose 13,900 ÷ 3500 = 4 pounds per week on The Final Diet.

As you approach your ideal weight, the drop in weight will slow down because your body size (weight) is getting closer to the body size (weight) that you are feeding on *The Final Diet*. Also the weight your body carries about the racquetball court will be smaller! (Fewer calories). You will gradually slim down to your ideal body weight. Keep up the great exercise–that really helps with your weight loss. You will become extremely fit (aerobic exercise). When you reach your ideal weight you can increase your intake slightly (say 500 calories/day) but keep your fat intake at about 20% of total calories. You will remain slim for life.

CHAPTER 15

MEAL PLANS—TWO WEEKS OF GREAT DINING!

We enjoyed writing this chapter. We created the recipes and we tried the delicious foods that are included in the 2 weeks of meal plans.

HOW TO USE THE MEAL PLANS:

- Follow the meal plans for the first 2 to 4 weeks. You can remain within your calorie and fat unit goals with very little effort. You will quickly learn how to use The Final Diet principles, making "smart substitutions." You will realize that you don't miss those nachos and chocolate chip cookies. You will learn the calorie and fat unit content of your favorite foods.

- We have chosen simple, filling, easy-to-prepare meals. All of the recipes are in the book—no meal will take over 15–20 minutes cooking time! The meal plans will give you *lots of food*—so hunger will not be a problem!

- Switch days, meals, foods at will—but achieve your calorie and fat unit goal every day. If you don't like a food (e.g. salmon)–substitute *or* pick another day or meal from the meal plans.

- If you fall off the wagon—climb back on!

- The meal plans are set for 1500 calories and 25–34 fat unit goals. They can easily be modified for greater or smaller goals. We'll use "day one" as an example. See table 15a.

TABLE 15A

DAY ONE - 1500 CALORIES / 24-34 FAT UNITS			
MEAL	**FOOD**	**CALORIES**	**FAT UNITS**
Breakfast	Raisin Bran 3/4 cup	115	1
	8 oz skim milk	85	0
	orange	65	0
	coffee	0	0
Snack	apple	80	1
Lunch	potato soup - 8 oz	110	0
	tuna sandwich	230	3
	skim milk - 8 oz	85	0
Snack	2 plums	70	1
Supper	salmon - 4 oz	220	12
	1 cup rice	240	1
	2 cups caesar salad	60	0
Dessert/ Snack	3.5 oz frozen yogurt	110	3
	TOTALS FOR THE DAY	1470	22

EXAMPLE A

Harry is 5'9" with an average build. Although he is now 190 pounds, he can now visualize his ideal body at 160 pounds (table 4a). His calorie goal is 2100 and his fat goal is 35–47 fat units (table 4c).

Looking at day one, Harry can take *an extra 600 calories and 11–23 fat units* over the meal plan (table 15a).

He has many options in selecting his extra calories and fat units.

		CALORIES	FAT UNITS
OPTION 1			
Add	1 extra tuna sandwich	230	3
	4 extra ounces salmon	*220*	*12*
	Total	450	15
OPTION 2			
Add	1 toast	70	0
	1 tbsp (Lite jam)	20	0
	3.5 oz extra frozen yogurt	110	3
	1 extra cup soup	110	0
	2 oz extra salmon	*220*	*12*
	Total	530	15
OPTION 3			
Add	1 extra cup rice	240	1
	1 extra tuna sandwich	*230*	*3*
	Total	470	4

The choices are endless. Harry can choose whatever extra foods he enjoys within his goals–as long as he knows what he is eating! (see food lists–chapter 17).

EXAMPLE B

Betty is just 5'1" with a small frame and ideal weight of 110 pounds (table 4a). She weighs 135 now and is determined to meet her final diet calorie goal of 1300 calories and her fat unit goal of 21–28 fat units (table 4b).

Looking at day one's plan (table 15a), Betty realized that *she must cut 200 calories and about 3 fat units* to reach her goal. She, too, has lots of options:

	SAVED CALORIES	SAVED FAT
OPTION 1		
Raisin Bran		
(*Reduce* 3/4 cup to ½ cup)	40	0
Salmon		
(*Reduce* 4 oz to 3 oz)	55	3
Eliminate Soup	*110*	*0*
Savings	195	3
OPTION 2		
Eliminate soup	110	0
Eliminate frozen yogurt	*110*	*3*
Savings	220	3

Again, Betty has many options. She also can bring in other foods from another day's menu plan–as long as she knows what she is eating.

- The meal plans are balanced to give the right proportion of carbohydrates (60%), protein (15%) and fat (15%). As you substitute, try to replace fruit with fruit and veggies with veggies, bread products with bread products...the meal plans will work very well for you.

- Take your calcium! Two 8 oz cups of skim milk and/or no fat yogurt will fill your daily need.

- *150 calorie desserts*
  We enclose a list of 21 fast, easy, delicious 150 calorie desserts (up to 3 fat units) on page 158 of the recipe section. When the meal plan specifies 150 calorie dessert, you can pick your favorite, or try a new dessert

from the list. We suggest that you save dessert until 8 or 9 in the evening as your evening snack.

- Drink six 8 oz glasses of ice water per day.

- *Meal proportions*
  Divide your daily food calories in the following way: breakfast 20%, lunch 25%, supper 40%, and snacks 15%. On a 1500 calorie diet, meals would be as follows: breakfast 300 calories, lunch 400 calories, supper 600 calories and snacks 200 calories.
  Dividing food this way, you won't experience hunger before meals *or* feel overly full after meals. You may reduce to 2 larger meals (e.g. brunch & supper on the weekends), or modify this suggestion to your life.

- After two weeks on the meal plan you will be educated and ready to plan your meals using the food lists (chapter 17), the recipes (chapter 16) and The Final Diet principles.

To make The Final Diet work for you

- Follow the meal plans on pages 83–90 for 2–4 weeks as you count calories and fat units.

- Count fat units *only* for 2–4 more weeks.

- Then make smart substitutions and follow the Final Diet principles *for life*. By making *smart substitutions* (chapter 9) and enjoying lots of complex carbohydrates (the Super Seven) we will spontaneously eat less than 20% of calorie as fat!

- We suggest you buy a calorie and fat counter handbook to help with your own meal planning and to supplement the food lists in this book (pg. 161–168).

"Fat and Cholesterol Counter" by the American Heart Association, 1991 is available at most book stores, or "The Complete Fat Counter" by Avery Publishing, 1992 New York.

Now on to two weeks of excellent, low fat dining!

1 fat unit = 1 gram of fat = 9 calories of fat

DAY 1 - (1500 CALORIES/25 FAT UNITS)			
MEAL	FOOD	CALORIES	FAT UNITS
Breakfast	Raisin Bran 3/4 cup	115	1
	8 oz skim milk	85	0
	orange	65	0
	coffee (black)	0	0
Snack	apple	80	1
Lunch	potato/onion soup (pg.113)	110	0
	tuna sandwich on whole wheat with tomato, lettuce, celery and mayo (pg.110)	230	3
	8 oz skim milk	85	0
Snack	2 plums	70	1
Supper	4 oz salmon steak or fillet in teriyaki sauce (pg.136)	220	12
	1 cup curried rice (pg.156)	240	1
	or vegetable rice (pg.156)		
	1 1/2 cups caesar salad (pg.118)	70	2
Dessert/ Snack	3.5 oz frozen yogurt	110	3
	TOTALS FOR THE DAY	1480	24

* this was a low fat day!! (about 12%) of calories

DAY 2 - (1500 CALORIES/25 FAT UNITS)			
MEAL	**FOOD**	**CALORIES**	**FAT UNITS**
Breakfast	8 oz skim milk	85	0
	3/4 cup no-fat yogurt &	85	0
	3/4 cup strawberries or 1/2 cup blueberries	30	0
	1 piece of toast with	60	0
	1 Tbsp. Ultra Light jam	20	0
	coffee (black)	0	o
Snack	2 peaches	75	0
Lunch	large whole wheat raisin bun (pg.95) with	230	2
	3 oz. chicken - (see Super Sandwich pg.100) with	120	4
	mustard, onion, tomato, lettuce, no-fat mayo	20	0
	1/2 cantaloupe	30	0
	diet drink	5	0
Snack	diet drink	1	0
Supper	Vegetarian Lasagna (pg.147)	320	12
	2 cups green salad with	50	0
	2 Tbsp. no fat dressing	30	0
	6 Triscuit Crackers with	120	4
	Salmon Dip (pg.105)	40	1
Dessert/ Snack	Choose a 150 calorie dessert (pg.158)	150	2
	TOTALS FOR THE DAY	1470	25

DAY 3 - (1500 CALORIES/25 FAT UNITS)			
MEAL	**FOOD**	**CALORIES**	**FAT UNITS**
Breakfast	Low fat veggie omelette (pg. 101)	130	6
	1 pieces raisin toast	70	1
	1 Tbsp. Ultra Light jam	20	0
	8 oz skim milk	85	0
	coffee	0	0
Snack	1 peach	45	0
Lunch	2 oz Chicken Super Sandwich (pg. 100) with whole wheat bun	250	6
	1 cup green grapes	60	0
	diet drink	1	0
Snack	1/2 cup no fat yogurt with blueberries	70	0
Supper	3 oz Pork Tenderloin (pg. 140)	250	6
	1/2 cup Cinnamon Applesauce (pg. 159)	26	0
	2 baked potato boats (pg. 154)	160	1
	Bean/Corn salad (pg. 116)	132	2
Dessert/ Snack	150 calorie dessert (pg. 158)	150	2
	TOTALS FOR THE DAY	1450	24

DAY 4 - (1500 CALORIES/25 FAT UNITS)			
MEAL	FOOD	CALORIES	FAT UNITS
Breakfast	Bran Crunchies - 3/4 cup	115	1
	6 oz skim milk	65	1
	1 cup fresh fruit	75	0
	coffee	0	0
Snack	1 apple	80	0
Lunch	Tuna/grape/peach/celery salad (pg. 123) with	100	4
	Whole wheat pita	106	1
	8 oz skim milk	87	0
Snack	1/2 cup frozen yogurt	110	3
Supper	1 cup Super Squash (pg. 150)	75	1
	1 cup long grain rice	210	2
	Chicken in Wine (pg. 134)	300	4
	Cucumber Salad (pg. 120)	40	0
Dessert/ Snack	150 calorie dessert (pg. 158)	150	3
	TOTALS FOR THE DAY	1513	20

* this was a low fat day!! (about 12%) of calories

DAY 5 - (1500 CALORIES/25 FAT UNITS)			
MEAL	FOOD	CALORIES	FAT UNITS
Breakfast	1 giant raisin whole wheat bun (pg. 95)	150	2
	2 Tbsp. Ultra Light Jam	40	0
	1 Banana	110	1
	8 oz skim milk	85	0
	coffee	0	0
Snack	1 orange	70	0
Lunch	Super Sandwich with 2 oz beef or ham (pg. 100)	150	10
	1 whole wheat raisin bun (pg. 95) with	150	2
	tomato, lettuce, onion, mustard, no-fat mayo	30	0
	1 apple	80	0
	diet drink	2	0
Snack	diet drink	2	0
Supper	Stir-fried shrimp (pg. 138) with pea pods	84	4
	1 cup Pasta (linguini)	210	3
	1 1/2 cup green salad with 2 Tbsp. no fat dressing	55	1
Dessert	1 cup no fat yogurt with	140	0
	1/2 cup grapes		
Snack	3 cups air popped popcorn	80	0
	TOTALS FOR THE DAY	1440	23

DAY 6 - (1500 CALORIES/25 FAT UNITS)

MEAL	FOOD	CALORIES	FAT UNITS
Breakfast	3/4 cup raisin bran	115	1
	1 cup strawberries	56	0
	1 piece whole wheat toast with	70	0
	1 Tbsp. Ultra Light jam	20	0
	8 oz skim milk	85	0
	coffee	0	0
Snack	Coffee	0	0
Lunch	1 cup no fat yogurt with	110	0
	1 cup green grapes	60	0
	1 whole wheat raisin bun (pg. 95) with	120	0
	1 Tbsp. Lite jam	30	0
	diet drink	1	0
Snack	1 plum	40	0
Supper	Stir-fried beef in ginger sauce (pg. 141)	375	20
	1 cup pasta	215	2
	Mandarin Orange salad with sweetened no-fat Italian dressing (pg. 120)	50	1
Dessert/ Snack	4 oz frozen blackcherry yogurt	130	2
	TOTALS FOR THE DAY	1480	26

DAY 7 (a weekend day) - (1500 CALORIES/25 FAT UNITS)

MEAL	FOOD	CALORIES	FAT UNITS
Breakfast	Low fat veggie omelette (pg. 101)	130	6
	2 pieces raisin whole wheat toast with	140	2
	2 Tbsp. Ultra Light jam	40	0
	8 oz skim milk	85	0
Snack			
Lunch	3/4 cup 1% cottage cheese	120	2
	1/2 cup unsweetened pineapple chunks	75	0
	1 toasted bagel with	160	2
	1 Tsp. Lite jam	30	0
Snack			
Supper	4 oz roast turkey or chicken (pg. 124)	160	8
	low fat yummy mashed potatoes (pg. 155)	210	0
	chicken broth gravy (pg. 125)	6	0
	1 cup cooked carrots	70	0
	1 1/2 cups green salad with 2 Tbsp. low fat dressing	55	1
	cranberry jello (pg. 125)	40	0
Dessert/ Snack	cantaloupe pieces with 3.5 oz. frozen yogurt	140	3
	TOTALS FOR THE DAY	1470	24

DAY 8 - (1500 CALORIES/25 FAT UNITS)			
MEAL	**FOOD**	**CALORIES**	**FAT UNITS**
Breakfast	3/4 cup raisin bran	115	1
	8 oz skim milk	85	0
	1 orange	65	0
	coffee	0	0
Snack	1 apple	80	0
Lunch	1 1/2 cups almond/chicken (turkey) salad (pg. 115)	190	8
	1 whole wheat raisin bun (pg. 95)	120	2
	1 apple	80	0
	diet drink	1	0
Snack	coffee	0	0
Supper	Turkey (chicken) Stroganoff (pg. 130) (1 serving)	400	10
	1 1/2 cups green beans	60	0
	1 1/2 cups green salad with 2 Tbsp. no fat dressing	55	1
Dessert/ Snack	1 cup no fat yogurt with 1/2 cup fresh raspberries	150	0
	TOTALS FOR THE DAY	1400	22

DAY 9 - (1500 CALORIES/25 FAT UNITS)			
MEAL	**FOOD**	**CALORIES**	**FAT UNITS**
Breakfast	8 oz skim milk	85	0
	3/4 cup no fat yogurt with	85	0
	3/4 cup strawberries or 1/2 cup blueberries	30	0
	1 piece toast	60	0
	1 Tbsp. Ultra Light jam	20	0
Snack	1 cup green grapes	60	0
Lunch	2 oz beef on rye super sandwich (pg. 100) with no fat mayo, mustard, lettuce, onion and tomato	320	12
	2 large dill pickles	40	0
	1 cup green grapes	60	0
	diet drink	1	0
Snack	coffee	0	0
Supper	2 cups Tuna Fettucini Delight (pg. 139)	350	6
	1 cup Bean Salad (pg. 117)	220	1
	1 whole wheat bun	120	2
Dessert/ Snack	1 peach	50	0
	TOTALS FOR THE DAY	1500	21

DAY 10 - (1500 CALORIES/25 FAT UNITS)			
MEAL	**FOOD**	**CALORIES**	**FAT UNITS**
Breakfast	1 large whole wheat raisin bun	150	2
	2 Tbsp. Ultra Light jam	40	0
	8 oz skim milk	85	0
	1/2 grapefruit	40	0
Snack	1 orange	65	0
Lunch	Pita pocket	110	1
	Tuna/grape/peach/celery salad (pg. 123)	100	1
	3.5 oz frozen yogurt	110	3
	8 oz skim milk	80	0
Snack	whole wheat raisin bun with	120	2
	1 Tbsp. Lite jam	30	0
Supper	1 1/2 cups chicken/rice/corn casserole (pg. 132)	360	7
	1 cup sweet 'n' sour onions (pg. 150)	50	0
	1 1/2 cups caesar salad (pg. 118)	40	0
Dessert/ Snack	150 calorie dessert (pg. 158)	150	3
	TOTALS FOR THE DAY	1530	19

DAY 11 - (1500 CALORIES/25 FAT UNITS)			
MEAL	**FOOD**	**CALORIES**	**FAT UNITS**
Breakfast	2 pieces french toast (pg. 102) with jam or catsup	210	2
	8 oz skim milk	85	0
	coffee	0	0
Snack	1 banana	100	1
Lunch	Super Sandwich with 2 oz ham	140	8
	mustard, no-fat mayo, lettuce, onion, tomato	20	0
	whole wheat bagel	160	2
Snack	1 large peach	45	0
Supper	Tomato & green bean chicken/turkey stirfry (pg.128)	300	7
	Curried brown rice (pg. 156)	240	1
	1 1/2 cups caesar salad (pg. 118)	40	0
Dessert/ Snack	1 cup no fat yogurt with 1/2 cup raspberries	150	2
	TOTALS FOR THE DAY	1470	23

DAY 12 - (1500 CALORIES/25 FAT UNITS)			
MEAL	FOOD	CALORIES	FAT UNITS
Breakfast	2 cups mixed fruit salad topped with	120	1
	1/4 cup no fat yogurt (and sweetener)	30	0
	8 oz skim milk	85	0
	1 piece whole wheat toast with Ultra Light jam	85	1
Snack	1 orange	70	0
Lunch	Super Sandwich (pg. 100) 3 oz chicken on	150	6
	2 slices whole wheat raisin bread with	220	2
	onion, tomato, no-fat mayo, mustard, lettuce	30	0
	1 1/2 cups green salad with 2 Tbsp. low fat dressing	60	1
Snack	1 apple	80	0
Supper	Salmon dip (pg. 105) with	60	3
	6 Ritz crackers	85	4
	8 oz Lentil-rice loaf (pg. 144)	180	1
	1 1/2 cups green salad with 2 Tbsp. low fat dressing	55	1
	Cucumber salad (pg. 120)	40	0
Dessert/ Snack	150 calorie dessert	150	3
	TOTALS FOR THE DAY	1500	23

DAY 13 - (1500 CALORIES/25 FAT UNITS)			
MEAL	FOOD	CALORIES	FAT UNITS
Breakfast	3/4 cup Bran Crunchies cereal	115	1
	8 oz skim milk	85	0
	1 cup blueberries	80	1
	coffee	0	0
Snack	1 plum	40	0
Lunch	1 1/2 cups 1% cottage cheese with 1/2 cup mixed fruit	180	3
	8 oz skim milk	85	0
	1 medium Whole Wheat Raisin Bun (pg. 95)	120	1
Snack			
Supper	Spaghetti with beef sauce (pg. 148)	230	14
	or (vegetarian spaghetti sauce - 80 cal/4 fat units)		
	1 cup noodles	160	1
	1 whole wheat bun with	120	2
	1 Tbsp. Ultra Light jam	20	0
	1 cup coleslaw (pg. 119) (side dish)	40	1
Dessert	1 1/2 cups green grapes	90	0
Snack	3 cups air popped popcorn	80	0
	TOTALS FOR THE DAY	1445	24

DAY 14 (a weekend day) - (1500 CALORIES/25 FAT UNITS)			
MEAL	**FOOD**	**CALORIES**	**FAT UNITS**
Breakfast	low fat omelette (pg. 101)	130	6
	2 pieces whole wheat toast	140	2
	2 Tbsp. Ultra Light jam	40	0
	8 oz skim milk	85	0
Snack			
Lunch	1 1/2 cups Cream of vegetable soup (pg. 110)	195	1
	1 whole wheat raisin bun (pg. 95)	120	2
	1 Tbsp. Ultra Light jam	20	0
	4 oz frozen yogurt	125	3
Snack	1 orange	60	0
Supper	4 oz Barbequed teriyaki turkey breast (pg. 124)	180	8
	1 cup curried rice (pg. 156)	170	1
	1 1/2 cups caesar salad (pg. 118)	40	0
	1 cup green beans	40	0
Dessert/ Snack	1 1/2 cups fresh fruit	120	0
	TOTALS FOR THE DAY	1465	23

(or repeat day 7 to have a turkey ready for week 3)

Chapter 16

The Final Diet—Recipes

Index of Recipes

1. Breads & muffins:

Honey & whole wheat bread with raisins	95
Whole wheat bread with herbs	96
Banana muffins	97
Pumpkin muffins	98
Zucchini muffins	99

2. Super sandwiches:

	100

3. Eggs:

Vegetable omelet	101
French toast	102

4. Appetizers:

Cottage cheese herb dip	103
Egg plant dip	104
Yogurt dip	104
Salmon dip	105
Veggie yogurt dip	105

5. Soups:

Beet soup	106
Butternut squash soup	107
Chilled creamed tomato soup	107
Chilled melon soup	108
Chilled peach strawberry soup	108
Cream of broccoli soup	109
Cream of vegetable soup	110
Fresh tomato & dill soup	110
Garden herb vegetable soup	111
Lentil tomato soup	112
Multi-bean soup	113
Potato and onion soup	113
Zucchini soup	114

6. Salads:

Almond chicken salad	115
Beans with corn salad	116
Bean salad	117
Caesar salad	118
Chicken rice salad	119
Coleslaw	119
Creamy cucumber salad	120
Green salad with mandarin sections	120
Mixed green salad	121
Pasta with green pea salad	121
Raspberry apple salad	122
Rice & pepper salad	122
Spinach rice salad	123
Tuna fruit salad	123

7. Main courses:

A. turkey

Grilled teriyaki turkey breasts	124
Roast turkey & trimmings	124/126
Spinach turkey loaf	127
Tomato & green bean turkey stir-fry	128
Turkey & rice casserole	129
Turkey Stroganoff	130

B. chicken

Apricot glazed chicken	131

Chicken breasts with ginger 131
Chicken & rice with corn casserole 132
Chicken & vegetable lasagna 133
Chicken in wine sauce 134
Tarragon & mustard baked chicken 135

C. SEAFOOD/FISH
Barbecued teriyaki salmon 136
Grilled salmon steaks 137
Shrimp & pea pod stir-fry 138
Tuna fettuccine delight 139

D. PORK
Apricot stuffed pork tenderloin 140

E. BEEF
Beef in ginger sauce 141
Spaghetti with meat sauce
(see veggie spaghetti pg. 148)

F. VEGETARIAN
Baked bean casserole 142
George's broccoli & garlic pasta 143
Lentil casserole 143
Lentils with rice loaf 144
Linguini with asparagus & red pepper 145
Vegetable chili 146
Vegetable lasagna 147
Veggie spaghetti 148

8. VEGETABLES:
Ratatouille 149
Sweet 'n sour onions 150
Super squash 150

9. POTATOES:
Dilled potato salad 151
Fresh basil & potato salad 151
New potatoes with cucumber dressing 152
Old-fashioned potato salad 153
Potato boats 154
Potatoes with yogurt 154
Yummy mashed potatoes 155

10. Rice:

Curried rice   156
Rice pudding   156
Vegetable rice   157

11. Desserts:

21 delicious low-fat desserts   158
Apple "Kelly"   159
Amy's cinnamon applesauce   159
Pears in red wine   160

1. BREAD & MUFFINS

HONEY & WHOLE WHEAT BREAD WITH RAISINS

Ingredients:

1½ tsp. yeast
2 tbsp. honey
2 cups warm water
½ cup raisins
5 cups whole wheat flour
1 cup white flour or omit white flour and use a total of 6 cups whole wheat flour
Pam vegetable spray

Method:

Combine yeast, honey and water; mix well. If using both white and whole wheat flour, combine and mix flours. Add raisins and 2 cups of flour mixture to yeast mixture; mix well. Add 2–3 cups more of flour mixture and mix. Pour mixture onto floured surface, knead and add flour as required. Knead until dough is elastic in nature but not sticky. Form into ball and place in a medium sized bowl that has been sprayed with Pam vegetable spray. Cover with cloth and let rise 2 hours or until dough has doubled in size. Then, knead down, divide in half, form loaves and place in 2 loaf pans that have been sprayed with Pam vegetable spray.
Cover and let rise 30–45 minutes.
Bake at 350°F for 20 minutes.

Makes 2 loaves of bread–110 calories, 1 fat unit per slice
or 24 small buns–110 calories, 1 fat unit per bun
or 18 medium buns–150 calories, 1.5 fat units per bun

WHOLE WHEAT BREAD WITH HERBS

Ingredients:

1 ½ tsp. yeast
2 tbsp. honey
2 cups warm water
1 tsp. dried dillweed
1 tsp. dried sweet basil
5 cups whole wheat flour
1 cup white flour
Pam vegetable spray

Method:

Combine yeast, honey and water; mix well. Add herbs to yeast mixture and mix well. Combine and mix flours. Stir in 2–3 cups of flour to yeast mixture. Pour mixture onto floured surface, knead and add flour as required (note: you may not need to add as much flour as directed). Knead until dough is elastic in nature but not sticky. Form into ball and place in a medium-sized bowl that has been sprayed with Pam vegetable spray. Cover with a clean, dry cloth and let rise 2 hours or until dough has doubled in size. Then, knead down, divide in half, form loaves and place in 2 loaf pans that have been sprayed with Pam. Cover and let rise 30–45 minutes. Bake at 375°F for 20 minutes.

Makes 2 loaves of bread–87 calories, .5 fat units per slice
Or 24 small buns–87 calories, .5 fat units per bun
Or 18 medium buns-150 calories, 1 fat unit per bun

BANANA MUFFINS

Ingredients:

½ cup unsweetened applesauce
½ cup white sugar
2 egg whites
1 tsp. Vanilla
1 tsp. Baking soda
½ cup no-fat yogurt
3 medium sized bananas, mashed
1 ½ cups flour
1 tsp. Cinnamon
Pam vegetable spray

Method:

Beat first 4 ingredients until light and fluffy. Dissolve baking soda in yogurt; add to batter and beat well. Lightly mix in mashed bananas. Add cinnamon and flour and stir until just mixed. Spray muffin pan with Pam. Bake at 350°F for 25 minutes.
Makes 12 medium sized muffins.
133 calories/muffin
1 fat units/muffin

PUMPKIN MUFFINS

Ingredients:

1 cup canned pumpkin
½ cup sugar
1 cup no-fat mayonnaise
2 cups flour
1 tsp. Baking soda
2 tsp. Baking powder
1 tsp. Pumpkin pie spice
Pam vegetable spray

Method:

Spray muffin tin with Pam vegetable spray. Whip together pumpkin, sugar and mayonnaise. Combine flour, baking soda, baking powder and pumpkin pie spice; mix well. Add flour mixture to pumpkin mixture; mix only until blended (do not over mix). Place mixture in muffin tin and bake at 400°F for 25-30 minutes.

Makes 12 medium size muffins
150 calories/muffin
1 fat unit/muffin

ZUCCHINI MUFFINS

Ingredients:

½ cup whole wheat flour
½ cup white flour
2 tsp. Baking powder
½ cup sugar
1 egg white
½ cup skim milk
½ cup zucchini, grated (or carrots)
Pam vegetable spray

Method:

Combine flours, baking powder and sugar; mix well. Beat egg white until foamy and add milk and zucchini. Add egg white and zucchini mixture to flour mixture. Stir just to moisten. Spray muffin tin with Pam vegetable spray. Fill cups. Bake at 375°F for 15–20 minutes.

Makes 8 muffins
120 calories/serving
1 fat unit/serving

2. SUPER SANDWICHES

		CALORIES	FAT UNITS
BREAD	2 pieces whole wheat bread	120	2
	2 pieces rye bread	120	2
	2 slices of Honey Whole Wheat Raisin bread	220	2
	1 Whole Wheat bun or homemade bun	120	1.5
FILLING	3 oz turkey breast	120	4.5
	3 oz chicken breast	150	6
	2 oz lean ham	140	8
	2 oz lean beef	150	8
	3 oz tuna & celery with no-fat mayonnaise	80	1
GARNISH	2 slices of tomato	10	0
	lettuce	2	0
	spanish onion	2	0
	1 Tbsp. no-fat mayonnaise	12	0
	2 tsp. mustard	10	0

MAKE UP A SANDWICH!!
WE SUGGEST A 300 CALORIE LIMIT FOR A 1500 CALORIE DIET.

3. EGGS

HIGH PROTEIN, LOW FAT, LOW CHOLESTEROL VEGETABLE OMELET

Ingredients:

1 whole egg
3 egg whites
½ cup skim milk
½ cup onion, chopped
½ cup green pepper, chopped
½ cup mushrooms, chopped
1½ tsp. Vegetable oil

Method:

Sauté vegetables in hot oil in non-stick pan until tender. Beat eggs; add milk. Add egg and milk mixture to vegetables in pan and cook until egg mixture thickens.
Serves 2

130 calories/serving
6 fat units/serving

French toast

Ingredients: (per serving)

3 egg whites
3 tbsp. Skim milk
1 tsp. vanilla flavoring
½ tsp. cinnamon
2 pieces whole wheat bread
Lite jam or catsup

Method:

Beat egg whites and skim milk in bowl and add cinnamon and vanilla. Soak bread in mixture until soggy. Cook in non-stick frying pan with Pam vegetable spray.

210 calories/serving
3 fat units/serving

4. APPETIZERS

COTTAGE CHEESE HERB DIP

Ingredients:

1 cup 1% cottage cheese
½ cup no-fat yogurt
1 green onion, chopped
½ tsp. garlic powder
½ tsp. celery seed
¼ tsp. dry mustard
¼ tsp. Worcestershire sauce
Pinch black pepper
Dash hot pepper sauce

Method:

Using a food processor or blender, process cottage cheese and yogurt until very smooth; stir in remainder of ingredients. Serve with raw vegetables.

Serves 6
40 calories/serving
1 fat unit/serving

EGGPLANT DIP

Ingredients:

1 medium sized eggplant
2 tbsp. fresh parsley, chopped
1 tbsp. olive oil
4 tsp. lemon juice
1 clove garlic, minced
1/4 tsp. salt
Pam vegetable spray

Method:

Heat oven to 400°F. Cut eggplant in half lengthwise and place cut side down in baking sheet that has been lightly sprayed with Pam vegetable spray; bake 45–50 minutes or until tender. When eggplant has cooled, peel and discard skin and process in food processor with chopping blade or mash. Add parsley, oil, lemon juice, garlic and salt; stir until just combined. Serve immediately or refrigerate to serve chilled.

Serves 8 (makes 2 cups)
25 calories/serving
1 fat unit/serving

YOGURT DIP

Ingredients:

½ cup no-fat yogurt
1 tbsp. chopped fresh parsley
1 tsp. dried dill weed
Dash of garlic powder

Method:

Combine above ingredients; refrigerate.

Serves 4
15 calories/serving
1 fat unit/serving

SALMON DIP

Ingredients:

1 (3 oz) can salmon, packed in water
1/4 cup onion and celery, finely chopped
2 tbsp. no-fat mayonnaise
1 tsp. low calorie sweetener

Method:

Drain salmon. Combine above ingredients; serve with Melba toast or Triscuit crackers.

Serves 6
120 calories/6 crackers
10 fat units

VEGGIE YOGURT DIP

Ingredients:

½ cup no-fat yogurt
1/4 tsp. dry mustard
1/4 head broccoli, leaves and stalks removed
2 tbsp. green onions
1/4 tsp. Thyme
1/4 tsp. Tarragon
Salt and pepper to taste
1 sprig parsley or 1 tbsp. chopped chives (optional)

Method:

Puree broccoli and onions together; mix together with remaining ingredients. Cover and refrigerate for several hours. Garnish with chives or parsley. Serve with raw vegetables.

Serves 4
20 calories/serving
0 fat units/serving

5. SOUPS

BEET SOUP

Ingredients:

1 tbsp. olive oil
1 medium sized onion, finely chopped
2 cloves garlic, minced
6–7 medium sized beets, cooked and sliced
1 can (14 oz) tomatoes
1 pkg. Beef stock with 1 cup water
2 tbsp. Apple cider vinegar
1 tsp. Caraway seed
Salt and pepper to taste
½ cup no-fat yogurt

Method:

In hot oil, sauté onion and garlic until tender. In large pot, bring to boil all ingredients except yogurt. Using a blender or food processor, puree beet mixture in batches until smooth. Return to pot and reheat. Garnish with swirls of yogurt.

Serves 6
110 calories/serving
1 fat unit/serving

BUTTERNUT SQUASH SOUP

Ingredients:

6 cups squash, peeled and cubed
3 cups chicken broth
1½ cups chopped onion
1 bay leaf
2 cloves garlic, chopped
1 tsp. nutmeg
Salt and pepper to taste

Method:

In large pot, combine squash, chicken broth, garlic, onions and bay leaf; bring to a boil. Cover, reduce heat and simmer until squash is tender (about 20 minutes) remove bay leaf. In blender or food processor, puree squash mixture in batches; season with herbs.

Serves 10
20 calories/cup
0 fat units/serving

CHILLED CREAMED TOMATO SOUP

Ingredients:

1½ cups no-fat yogurt
1 tbsp. tomato paste
1½ cups tomato juice
½ cup English cucumber, peeled and chopped
2 tbsp. green onion, finely chopped
2 tbsp. Lemon juice
½ tbsp. fresh chives, chopped
Salt and pepper to taste
4 slices lemon (optional)

Method:

Combine yogurt and tomato paste; mix well. Add remaining ingredients, except chives and lemon slices. Stir, cover and refrigerate for 1–2 hours. Garnish with chives and lemon slices.

Serves 4
95 calories/serving
0 fat units/serving

CHILLED MELON SOUP

Ingredients:

1 ripe cantaloupe, cut into wedges with seeds and peel removed
1 cup no-fat yogurt
3 tbsp. lemon juice
½ tsp. fresh ginger root or 1/4 tsp. dried
2 tbsp. fresh mint leaves, chopped

Method:

Using a blender or food processor, puree cantaloupe; add yogurt, lemon juice and ginger. Process to mix. Refrigerate until serving. Garnish with fresh mint.

Serves 4
55 calories/serving
0 fat units/serving

CHILLED PEACH STRAWBERRY SOUP

Ingredients:

2 peaches, peeled and sliced or 1 nectarine sliced
1½ cups strawberries, sliced
1½ cups no-fat yogurt
1 tbsp. granulated brown low calorie sweetener
1 tbsp. lemon juice
Lemon slices
Fresh mint sprigs

Method:

Using a food processor with metal blade or blender, combine all ingredients except lemon slices and mint; process until smooth. Pour into medium sized bowl; cover and refrigerate 1–2 hours. Spoon into soup bowls. Garnish with lemon slices and mint.

Serves 4 (1 cup serving)
80 calories/serving
1 fat unit/serving

CREAM OF BROCCOLI SOUP

Ingredients:

6 cups broccoli, with leaves removed and coarsely chopped
8 medium sized potatoes, peeled and quartered
1 medium sized onion, sliced
3 pkgs. chicken broth, without water added
1/4 tsp. garlic salt
½ tsp. curry (optional)
Salt and pepper to taste

Method:

Cook broccoli, potatoes and onions until well cooked. Retain all cooking juices. Using a food processor, with chopping blade, process broccoli mixture until pureed, adding cooking juices and water as required, to make a thick consistency. Add chicken broth and herbs and more water, if required. Bring to a slow boil. Serve immediately.

Serves 8
150 calories/serving
1 fat unit/serving

CREAM OF VEGETABLE SOUP

Ingredients:

4 medium sized potatoes, diced
2 cups diced carrots
1 cup onion, finely chopped
3 cloves garlic, finely chopped
2 pkgs. chicken broth
1 cup water
3 cups skim milk
1 tsp. nutmeg
1 tsp. basil
Salt and pepper to taste

Method:

Cook vegetables and garlic in chicken broth and water until vegetables are slightly softened. With heat turned down to low, add milk and herbs. Heat until mixture is hot; serve immediately.

Serves 6
155 calories/serving
1 fat unit/serving

FRESH TOMATO AND DILL SOUP

Ingredients:

3–4 large tomatoes
½ cup no-fat yogurt
1 tbsp. dried dill weed
2 tbsp. green onion, chopped
Salt and pepper to taste

Method:

Using a blender or food processor, puree tomatoes; add yogurt and herbs and puree until smooth. Stir in onions. Cover and refrigerate for 2–3 hours. Serve chilled.

Serves 4
45 calories/serving
0 fat units/serving

GARDEN HERB VEGETABLE SOUP

Ingredients:

2 pkgs. chicken broth with 2 cups water
1 cup chopped tomatoes
4 medium sized potatoes, quartered
½ cup fresh green beans, cut into 2" pieces
1 can (6 oz) tomato paste
2 tbsp. fresh parsley, chopped
1 tbsp. dried dill weed
2 tbsp. fresh chives or green onions, chopped

Method:

Combine all ingredients, except chives or onions. Bring to a boil; reduce heat; cover and simmer for 30 minutes or until vegetables are tender. Serve immediately. Garnish with chives or green onion.

Serves 5
150 calories/serving
1 fat unit/serving

LENTIL TOMATO SOUP

Ingredients:

1 whole head garlic, minced
4 carrots, thinly sliced
2 stalks celery, finely chopped
1 medium sized onion, finely chopped
6 cups chicken broth
1 can (28 oz) plum tomatoes, chopped with juice
½ cup green lentils
½ cup macaroni
2 small zucchini, thinly sliced
1/4 cup fresh parsley, chopped
Salt and pepper to taste
6 small sprigs fresh parsley (optional)

Method:

Combine all ingredients, except macaroni, zucchini and parsley. Bring to a boil, reduce heat and simmer covered for 20 minutes. Add macaroni and simmer for an additional 15 minutes. Then stir in zucchini and parsley; simmer until zucchini is tender (about 5 minutes). Serve immediately. Garnish with fresh parsley sprigs.

Serves 7
110 calories/serving
2 fat units/serving

MULTI–BEAN SOUP
(COMBINATION OF PEAS, LENTILS, BARLEY AND RICE)

Ingredients:

1 cup dry soup mix (Loretta brand)–multi bean soup mix
1 pkg. chicken broth
1 medium size onion, finely chopped
6 cups boiling water
1 bay leaf
Salt and pepper to taste
½ tsp. dried sweet basil

Method:

Combine soup mix and water; bring to a boil then simmer uncovered until ingredients soften (about 45 minutes). Add onion, broth and spices; simmer until onion is tender. Remove bay leaf before serving.

Serves 4
70 calories/serving
1 fat unit/serving

POTATO & ONION SOUP

Ingredients:

4 medium sized potatoes, diced
1 medium sized onion, diced
2 cloves garlic, finely chopped
2 pkgs. chicken broth
3 cups water
1 tsp. dried dill weed
2 tsp. parsley
Salt and pepper to taste

Method:

Combine vegetables, garlic, pkgs. of chicken broth and water; bring to full boil; reduce heat, add herbs and simmer until vegetables are tender.

Makes 4 cups
110 calories/cup
0 fat units/cup

ZUCCHINI SOUP

Ingredients

8 small zucchini, peeled and chopped
½ tbsp. olive oil
1 leek, chopped
4 cups chicken broth
½ cup dry white wine
2 tsp. tarragon or 2 tbsp. fresh and chopped
2 tbsp. fresh parsley, finely chopped
1 tbsp. chives, chopped
1 tbsp. grated lemon rind

Method:

Sauté leek in hot oil until tender. Steam zucchini until tender; retaining cooking juice. Using a blender or food processor, puree leek and zucchini until smooth, adding cooking juice and chicken broth as necessary. Return mixture to saucepan; add wine and remainder of chicken broth; season with herbs. Cover and simmer for 5 minutes. Serve immediately. Garnish with lemon rind and mixture of herbs.

Serves 8
50 calories/serving
1 fat unit/serving

6. Salads

Almond chicken salad

Ingredients:

2 cups cooked turkey or chicken breast, cooled, then cubed
1 cup pea pods, cut in half diagonally and blanched
1 cup cubed, seedless cucumber
3/4 cup celery, chopped
1 medium sized apple, unpeeled and chopped
1/4 cup sliced green onions
1 tsp. lemon juice
1/8 tsp. pepper
½ cup no-fat mayonnaise
1 oz. slivered almonds, toasted (optional)

Method:

Pour lemon juice over chopped apple. In large bowl, combine all ingredients except almonds; toss lightly. Cover and refrigerate. Prior to serving, garnish with almonds.

Serves 4 (1½ cup serving)
190 calories/serving
8 fat units/serving

BEANS WITH CORN SALAD

Ingredients:

4 cups fresh green beans, trimmed and cooked until tender
2 cups whole baby corn cobs, cooked until tender
½ cup green onions, thinly sliced
1/4 cup white wine vinegar
2 tbsp. dijon mustard
2 tbsp. honey
1 tsp. ground dried gingerroot
½ cup no-fat Italian dressing
Salt and pepper to taste

Method:

Drain vegetables well; cover and refrigerate 1–2 hours. Combine vinegar, mustard, honey, ginger root, dressing and salt and pepper; mix well. Before serving, lightly toss dressing with vegetable mixture.

Serves 6
135 calories/serving
1 fat unit/serving

BEAN SALAD

Ingredients:

2 cups lima beans
2 cups kidney beans
2 cups green beans
1 cup yellow beans
1 medium sized Spanish onion, thinly sliced
1 cup green pepper, finely chopped
4 tbsp. low calorie sweetener
½ cup wine vinegar
½ cup no-fat Italian dressing
1 tsp. salt
½ tsp. dry mustard
½ tsp. crumbled tarragon
½ tsp. basil
2 tbsp. fresh parsley, chopped

Method:

Combine beans, onion and green pepper; set aside. In large jar with lid, combine sweetener, vinegar, Italian dressing, and herbs; shake well. Pour combined dressing over bean mixture; marinate over night, stirring once or twice. Before serving, stir and drain well.

Serves 10
135 calories/serving
1 fat unit/serving

CAESAR SALAD (A WINNER!)

Ingredients:

1 med. bunch romaine lettuce
⅓ cup no-fat mayonnaise
1 tsp. dijon mustard
1 tsp. Worcestershire sauce
2 cloves garlic, crushed
3–4 tbsp. vinegar
Salt and pepper to taste
Sweetener (low calorie) to taste

Method:

Combine mayo, mustard, Worcestershire sauce, garlic and salt and pepper; mix well; stir in vinegar. Sweeten to taste with sweetener. Add to lettuce shreds. Croutons, mushrooms and shrimp optional.

Serves 5 (1 ½ cups)
40 calories/serving
0 fat units/serving

CHICKEN RICE SALAD

Ingredients:

3 cups cubed cooked chicken breast
2 cups cooked long-grain brown rice
1/4 cup green bell pepper, chopped
1/4 cup green onions, sliced
1 (20 oz) can chunk pineapple, drained
1/4 cup slivered toasted almonds
½ cup no-fat Italian dressing
1 tsp. sweetener
1/4 tsp. tarragon
Salt and pepper to taste

Method:

Combine dressing, sweetener, tarragon and salt and pepper; mix well and set aside. Combine chicken, brown rice, green pepper and onions. Add dressing and toss gently; cover and refrigerate for several hours. Before serving, fold in pineapple and almonds.

Serves 6–8
300 calories/serving
8 fat units/serving

COLESLAW

Ingredients:

½ cup no-fat mayonnaise
1/4 cup no-fat yogurt
2 tbsp. vinegar
4 tsp. low calorie sweetener
2½ cups shredded white cabbage
½ cup grated carrot
½ cup diced green pepper

Method:

Combine mayo, yogurt, vinegar and sweetener. Add vegetables; toss lightly.

Serves 4
40 calories/serving
1 fat unit/serving

CREAMY CUCUMBER SALAD

Ingredients:

2 cups thinly sliced cucumber (with skin on)
1 medium onion, very thinly sliced
½ tsp. salt
¼ cup vinegar
½ cup no-fat yogurt
2 tsp. dried dill weed
½ tsp. sweetener
¼ tsp. pepper

Method:

Combine salt, vinegar, yogurt, dill, sweetener and pepper; mix well. Add to sliced cucumber and onion.

Serves 4
40 calories/serving
0 fat units/serving

GREEN SALAD WITH MANDARIN SECTIONS

Ingredients:

¼ head lettuce
¼ bunch romaine
2 medium stalks celery, diced
2 green onions, chopped finely
1 can (11 oz) mandarin orange sections, drained
¼ cup no-fat Italian dressing
2 tbsp. low calorie sweetener
2 tbsp. vinegar
1 tbsp. fresh snipped parsley
Dash red pepper sauce
Salt and pepper to taste

Method:

Combine dressing, sweetener, vinegar and spices in tightly covered jar; shake well and refrigerate. Combine lettuces, celery, onion and orange sections. Just prior to serving, add dressing to lettuce mixture.

Serves 4
50 calories/serving
2 fat units/serving

MIXED GREEN SALAD

Ingredients:

1 head lettuce
½ cup celery, chopped
¼ cup onion, finely chopped
¼ cup mushrooms, finely sliced
¼ cup carrots, chopped
¼ cup green pepper, chopped
1 medium sized tomato, chopped
2 tbsp. no-fat Ranch or French or Italian dressing per serving
Salt and pepper to taste

56 calories/serving
1 fat unit/serving

PASTA WITH GREEN PEA SALAD

Ingredients:

4 cups small shell macaroni, cooked
2 (19 oz) cans green peas, drained
3 stalks celery, finely chopped
1 red apple, chopped
1 tsp. lemon juice
¾ cup no-fat mayonnaise
1 tbsp. vinegar
2 tsp. low calorie sweetener
Salt and pepper to taste

Method:

Drain macaroni and rinse with cold water. Sprinkle lemon juice over chopped apple. Combine macaroni, peas, celery and apple. In separate container, combine mayonnaise, vinegar, sweetener and salt and pepper; mix well and combine with macaroni mixture.

Serves 6 (1 cup servings)
205 calories/serving
2 fat units/serving

RASPBERRY APPLE SALAD

Ingredients:

2 pkgs. Lite Jello, raspberry flavored
2 cups boiling water
1 cup cold water
1 can (19 oz) apple sauce, unsweetened

Method:

Combine Jello with boiling water; stir well; add cold water and stir. Add apple sauce; pour into mold and chill for several hours. Good with pork tenderloin.

Serves 10
26 calories/serving
1 fat unit/serving

RICE AND PEPPER SALAD

Ingredients:

1½ cups long-grain brown rice, cooked as directed
½ cup no-fat mayonnaise
1 tbsp. fresh parsley, chopped
½ tsp. thyme
½ tsp. basil
1 tsp. lemon juice
1 small sweet red pepper, finely chopped
1 small green pepper, finely chopped
¼ cup green onion, chopped
Salt and pepper to taste

Method:

Chill rice; add peppers. Combine mayonnaise, herbs and lemon juice; mix well. Combine with rice and pepper mixture. Garnish with green onions.

Serves 4
90 calories/serving
1 fat unit/serving

SPINACH RICE SALAD

Ingredients:

1 cup long-grain brown rice, cooked
½ cup no-fat Italian dressing
1 tbsp. soy sauce
1 tsp. low calorie sweetener
1 clove garlic, minced
Salt and pepper to taste
2 cups fresh spinach, cut into medium-sized pieces
½ cup celery, thinly sliced
¼ cup green onion, chopped
¼ cup red pepper, finely chopped
½ cup mushrooms, finely sliced

Method:

Combine dressing, soy sauce, sweetener, garlic and salt and pepper; mix well and stir into warm rice. Cover and refrigerate 1–2 hours. Before serving, combine with remaining ingredients; toss gently.

Serves 4
100 calories/serving
1 fat unit/serving

TUNA FRUIT SALAD

Ingredients:

2 cans (6.5 oz) tuna, (packed in water), drained
2 cups celery, diced
1 orange, chopped
2 peaches, chopped
2 cups seedless grapes, sliced in half
½ cup no-fat mayonnaise
Salt and pepper to taste
1 tsp. Thyme

Method:

Combine tuna and fruit; add mayo and herbs and toss lightly.

Serves 6
135 calories/serving (1¼ cups)
1 fat unit/serving

7. MAIN COURSES

A. TURKEY

GRILLED TERIYAKI TURKEY BREASTS

Ingredients:

¼ cup soy sauce
½ tbsp. honey
1 clove garlic, minced
½ tbsp. fresh ginger root, finely chopped or ½ tsp. ground ginger
2 oz. white wine or apple juice
6 (4 oz each) turkey breasts

Method:

Combine all ingredients, except turkey; mix well. Place turkey in shallow dish; pour soy sauce mixture over turkey and marinate for several hours, turning turkey several times. Drain marinade. Grill or barbecue turkey breasts until tender.

Serves 6
180 calories/serving
8 fat units/serving

ROAST TURKEY & TRIMMINGS

We suggest choosing a turkey that does not have butter added. Utility turkey is good, if you don't mind a missing wing or leg. Completely remove skin and visible fat from the bird with sharp knife and scissors.

Sprinkle cavity and exterior of turkey liberally with mixture of herbs: thyme, sage and black pepper. A roasting pan with a rack is ideal, as it allows the fatty juices to drain off. Cook as directed (see turkey page 43)

240 calories/6 oz serving
12 fat units/6 oz serving

THE TRIMMINGS:

1. CRANBERRY JELLO

Ingredients:

1 pkg. Diet Jello
1 cup whole berry cranberry sauce

Method:

Make up Jello as directed; add cranberry sauce; mix and refrigerate.

Serves 12
40 calories/serving
0 fat units/serving

2. CHICKEN BROTH GRAVY

Ingredients:

1 cube or pkg. Chicken broth
1 cup water
1 tbsp. cornstarch

Method:

Mix ingredients and heat until boiling with frequent stirring. Simmer in pot.

Serves 6
6 calories/serving
0 fat units/serving

3. TURKEY STUFFING

Ingredients:

4 slices low-fat bread
1 small onion, finely chopped
½ cup celery, finely chopped
1 medium sized apple, cored and diced
¼ cup apple juice
1 tsp. thyme
1 tsp. sage
Salt and pepper to taste

Method:

Cube bread slices and combine all ingredients; mix lightly and stuff cavity of turkey loosely.

Serves 8
55 calories/serving
1 fat unit/serving

SPINACH TURKEY LOAF

Ingredients:

1½ lbs. ground raw turkey
½ cup onion, diced
½ cup carrot, shredded
½ cup uncooked oatmeal
½ cup no-fat yogurt
½ tsp. dried parsley
½ tsp. sage
½ tsp. thyme
½ tsp. ground black pepper
2 egg whites, slightly beaten
1 pkg (10 oz) frozen chopped spinach, thawed
3 tbsp. no-fat mayonnaise
½ tsp. Nutmeg
Pam vegetable spray
Fresh parsley (optional)

Method:

Combine turkey, onion, carrot, oatmeal, yogurt, sage, thyme, parsley and black pepper in a large bowl; stir in egg whites. Drain spinach well and combine with mayonnaise and nutmeg. Set aside. Spray 9x5x3 loaf pan with Pam. Spoon half of turkey mixture into pan, then spread entire spinach mixture in a 2" wide strip down center of turkey layer, leaving a ½" space at ends of pan. Spoon remaining turkey mixture over spinach layer. Bake uncovered at 350°F for approximately 1 hour. Slice to serve and garnish with fresh parsley.

Serves 8
130 calories/serving
3 fat units/serving

TOMATO AND GREEN BEAN TURKEY STIR-FRY

Ingredients:

16 oz turkey, cooked and coarsely chopped
1 medium sized onion, coarsely chopped
1 cup green pepper, coarsely chopped
½ cup red pepper, coarsely chopped
1 cup fresh green beans, lightly steamed
1 medium sized zucchini, sliced
3 medium sized field tomatoes, coarsely chopped
3 cloves garlic, finely chopped
2 tbsp. vegetable oil
4 tbsp. soy sauce
1 pkg. chicken broth with ½ cup water
Salt and pepper to taste
½ tsp. ground ginger

Method:

Combine soy sauce, chicken broth and herbs; set aside. Sauté onions, peppers, zucchini and garlic in hot oil until tender. Add turkey pieces, beans and tomatoes. Add soy sauce mixture and stir until thickened. Cover and simmer for 5 minutes. Serve immediately with pasta or rice.

Serves 4
300 calories/serving
7 fat units/serving

TURKEY AND RICE CASSEROLE

Ingredients:

2 cups long-grain brown rice
3 cups boiling water
3 pkgs. chicken broth
3 tbsp. soy sauce
1 cup celery, finely chopped
1½ cups mushrooms, sliced
1 medium sized onion, finely chopped
1½ cups green pepper, finely chopped
2 cups left-over small pieces turkey
1 tbsp. olive oil

Method:

Mix all ingredients together in large casserole dish. Bake, covered at 350°F for 1½ hours.

Serves 4
280 calories/serving
5 fat units/serving

Turkey stroganoff

Ingredients:

1 medium onion, diced
1 small can of button mushrooms
4 (4 oz) chicken or turkey breasts
4 cups cooked eggless noodles (8 oz dry pasta)
½ cup no-fat yogurt
1 pkg. Chicken broth dissolved in 1 cup water
2 tbsp. Cornstarch
2 tsp. Thyme
½ tsp. ground black pepper
1 tsp. canola oil
Fresh parsley (optional)

Method:

Microwave the thawed skinless, boneless chicken breasts on high power for 5 minutes or bake in oven until cooked. Cool and cut into ½ " wide strips. Mix cornstarch, thyme and pepper with chicken broth. Sauté onions in 1 tsp. of oil in non-stick pan. Add mushrooms and chicken to pan to lightly brown; then add chicken broth mixture to the onion, mushroom and chicken mixture in the pan and simmer until thickened. Just before serving, stir in the no-fat yogurt. Serve over noodles and garnish with parsley.

Serves 4
400 calories/serving
10 fat units/serving

B. CHICKEN

APRICOT GLAZED CHICKEN

Ingredients:

4 (4 oz) chicken breasts, boned and skinned
2 tbsp. sugar-reduced apricot jam
2 tbsp. unsweetened orange juice
1 clove garlic, minced
2 tsp. soy sauce
1 tsp. ground ginger
½ tsp. dry mustard

Method:

Combine all ingredients, except chicken; mix well. Spoon over chicken and bake, covered at 350°F for 35 minutes. Remove cover, baste with sauce and bake 10 minutes longer.

Serves 4
230 calories/serving
6 fat units/serving

CHICKEN BREASTS WITH GINGER

Ingredients:

4 (4 oz) chicken breasts boned and skinned
1 small onion, finely chopped
2 garlic cloves, minced
1 tsp. ground ginger
2 tbsp. soy sauce
1 tbsp. dry sherry
2 tsp. Honey

Method:

Combine all ingredients, except chicken; mix well and pour over chicken. Marinate for at least 1 hour or overnight, turning a few times. Bake, covered at 350°F for 20 minutes. Remove cover and bake 10 minutes longer.

Serves 4
230 calories/serving
6 fat units/serving

CHICKEN & RICE WITH CORN CASSEROLE

Ingredients:

4 cups long-grain brown rice, cooked
1 cup frozen or canned kernel corn
4 (4 oz each) chicken breasts, boneless and skinless
½ cup no-fat mayonnaise
2 tsp. soy sauce
½ cup onions, coarsely chopped
½ cup green or red pepper, coarsely chopped
½ cup mushrooms, coarsely chopped
½ tsp. tarragon
Salt and pepper to taste
1 tbsp. vegetable oil
½ tsp. sweet basil

Method:

Microwave chicken on high for 5 minutes or bake in oven until pinkness has disappeared; cool, then cut into cubes. Sauté onions and peppers in hot oil in non-stick pan. Remove from pan, then sauté mushrooms in same pan. Combine all ingredients in casserole dish. One half hour before serving, heat casserole in 350°F oven.

Serves 6
360 calories/cup
7 fat units/cup

CHICKEN AND VEGETABLE LASAGNA (EXCELLENT!)

Ingredients:

½ lb. lean ground cooked chicken or turkey
½ cup onion, chopped
2 garlic cloves, minced
1 can (28 oz) tomatoes
1 can (5½ oz) tomato paste
¾ cup water
4 medium carrots, diced
1 bunch broccoli, chopped
½ lb. mushrooms, sliced
¼ cup fresh parsley, chopped
¾ lb. lasagna noodles
1 pkg (6 oz) low-fat cheese, grated or sliced
Salt and pepper to taste
Pam vegetable spray

Method:

In Teflon pan sprayed with vegetable spray, sauté onions and garlic; add tomatoes, tomato paste, water and salt and pepper. Cook, uncovered for 15 minutes; add vegetables, chicken and parsley. Cook, covered on low heat for about 30 minutes. Cook lasagne according to package directions. Spoon of sauce into 13x9" baking dish. Place ⅓ of noodles over sauce. Repeat layers twice, ending with sauce. Top with cheese. Bake covered at 350°F for 30 minutes. Let stand 10 minutes before serving.

Serves 8
340 calories/serving
9 fat units/serving

Chicken in wine sauce (excellent!)

Ingredients:

4 (4 oz) chicken breasts, cooked and cubed
2 (8 oz) pkgs. Mushrooms
1 pkg. chicken broth
½ cup orange juice
½ cup dry white wine
4 carrots, sliced julienne style
½ cup skim milk
1 tbsp. granulated brown low-calorie sweetener
Salt and pepper to taste
Pam vegetable spray (2 sec)
1 tbsp. cornstarch

Method:

Use food processor or finely chop 1 pkg. mushrooms; add skim milk. In a small pot, combine mushroom mixture, chicken broth, orange juice, wine, sweetener, salt and pepper, and cornstarch; mix well. Simmer until thickened. Place carrots in casserole dish; add mushroom mixture. Add chicken to mixture but do not stir in.

Spray Teflon coated pan with Pam spray; heat and sauté 1 pkg. sliced mushrooms until lightly browned. Add to casserole dish but do not stir in. Cover and bake at 350°F for 45 minutes.

Serves 4
300 calories/serving
4 fat units/serving

TARRAGON AND MUSTARD BAKED CHICKEN

Ingredients:

2 tbsp. honey
2 tbsp. dijon mustard
1 tbsp. lemon juice
1 tsp. dried tarragon
2 cloves garlic, minced
4 (4 oz) chicken breasts, with skin and bone removed
Lemon slices (optional)
Pam vegetable spray

Method:

Combine first 5 ingredients; mix well. Place chicken in baking pan sprayed with Pam. Spread mustard mixture over chicken and bake, covered at 350°F for 30 minutes. Remove lid and bake 10 minutes longer. Garnish with lemon slices.

Serves 4
220 calories/serving
2 fat units/serving

C. Seafood/fish

Barbecued teriyaki salmon

Ingredients:

1⁄4 cup soy sauce
1⁄4 cup dry sherry
1 tbsp. honey
2 cloves garlic, minced
1 tsp. ground ginger (or 1 tbsp. fresh chopped ginger root)
½ tsp. black pepper
4 salmon steaks
* thin strips of peeled cucumber (optional)

Method:

Combine all ingredients except salmon and cucumber. Place salmon in shallow dish; pour soy sauce mixture over salmon; cover and refrigerate for several hours, turning salmon several times.

Brush marinade over salmon while grilling or cooking on barbecue. Serve immediately. Garnish with cucumber strips.

Serves 4
220 calories/serving
12 fat units/serving

GRILLED SALMON STEAKS

Ingredients:

½ cup no-fat yogurt
1 tbsp. olive oil
1 tbsp. lime juice
1 tsp. honey
1 tbsp. fresh ginger root, minced or 1 tsp. ground ginger
2 cloves garlic, minced
Salt and pepper to taste
4 (4 oz) salmon steaks
Lime wedges (optional)

Method:

Combine all ingredients, except salmon and lime wedges; mix well. Place salmon in shallow dish; add yogurt mixture. Cover and marinade in fridge several hours, turning salmon 4–5 times. Grill salmon (on lightly oiled grill) over medium high heat until tender. Brush salmon with additional marinade while grilling. Garnish with lime wedges.

Serves 4
255 calories/serving
15 fat units/serving

SHRIMP AND PEA POD STIR-FRY (EXCELLENT!)

Ingredients:

2 tbsp. soy sauce
1 tsp. dried ginger
¼ cup red wine
¼ cup wine vinegar
1½ tsp. cornstarch
1 tbsp. no-fat Italian dressing
1 cup mushrooms, sliced
1 clove garlic, minced
1 lb. shrimp, shelled, deveined and cooked
3 cups pea pods

Method:

Combine soy sauce, ginger, wine, vinegar and cornstarch; set aside. Heat dressing in teflon skillet; add mushrooms and sauté until lightly browned; stir in garlic; add shrimp. Sauté for a few minutes; add pea pods and soy sauce mixture. Cook, stirring constantly, until pods turn bright green and sauce comes to a boil. Serve immediately. Serve with pasta or rice.

Serves 4
120 calories/serving (before pasta or rice)
1 fat unit/serving

TUNA FETTUCCINE DELIGHT

Ingredients:

4 cups (8 oz dry) fettuccine noodles
2 medium sized onions, coarsely chopped
4 medium sized zucchini, coarsely chopped
1 tbsp. olive oil
1 tsp. dried dill weed
1 tsp. curry powder
1½ cups no-fat yogurt
2 (6 oz) cans tuna, packed in water
Salt and pepper to taste

Method:

Cook fettuccine as per package directions. In large pan, sauté onions and zucchini in hot oil until tender; add herbs. Add tuna and yogurt; stir and cook just until heated through. Toss lightly with pasta. Serve immediately.

Serves 4
350 calories/serving
6 fat units/serving

D. Pork

Apricot stuffed pork tenderloin

Ingredients:

¼ cup dried currants
¼ cup dried apricots, finely chopped
2 tbsp. bourbon
1 tbsp. water
1 lb. boneless pork tenderloin
1 cup low-fat bread cubes
1/4 cup celery, finely chopped
½ tsp. rosemary
½ tsp. sage
Salt and pepper to taste
1 egg white, lightly beaten

Method:

Soak dried fruit in bourbon and water. Cut tenderloin lengthwise down center but not all the way through. Pound between 2 sheets of waxed paper until tenderloin is an even 1/4" thickness. Combine bread cubes, herbs, egg white and fruit mixture; mix well. Spread bread mixture down center of tenderloin leaving ½" on either end. Bring up long sides of tenderloin to enclose filling, overlapping long edges slightly. Secure with string every few inches. Arrange on rack in roasting pan. Bake at 400°F for 50 minutes. Let stand 5 minutes before serving.

Serves 4
230 calories/serving
8 fat units/serving

E. Beef

Beef in ginger sauce stir-fry

Ingredients:

1 cup tomato juice
3 tbsp. soy sauce
½ tsp. ground ginger
1 tbsp. cornstarch
1 tbsp. granulated brown low calorie sweetener
5 drops hot pepper sauce
1 lb. beef, flank portion, cooked and cut into 1/8" strips
1½ cups onion, quartered
1 cup green pepper, coarsely chopped
1 cup red pepper, coarsely chopped
2 small zucchini, sliced
1/4 cup chicken broth

Method:

Combine first 6 ingredients; mix well and set aside. Heat chicken broth in pan; steam vegetables until tender; add beef and tomato juice mixture. Cook until heated through. Serve immediately. Serve with pasta or rice.

Serves 4
375 calories/serving
20 fat units/serving

F. VEGETARIAN

BAKED BEAN CASSEROLE

Ingredients:

2 cups dried white beans (8 cups cooked beans)
1 ½ tsp. dry mustard
1 tsp. salt
1 tsp. pepper
1 medium sized onion, finely chopped
4 tbsp. brown sugar sweetener
2 tbsp. molasses

Method:

Rinse beans and soak overnight in cold water or cover with cold water, boil for 2 minutes, remove from heat, cover and let stand 1 hour; drain. Cover again with cold water. Bring to a boil, reduce heat and simmer, covered for 40 minutes. Drain beans, reserving liquid. Transfer beans to a heavy casserole pot; stir in mustard, salt and pepper and onion. Stir in sufficient amount of reserved liquid to top beans. Cover and bake at 350°F for 5 hours, stirring occasionally and adding more liquid if necessary. 1 hour before serving, remove lid and allow beans to brown. 30 minutes before serving, stir in remaining ingredients.

Serves 8
270 calories/serving
1 fat units/serving

GEORGE'S BROCCOLI & GARLIC PASTA

Ingredients:

1½ tbsp. olive oil
4 garlic cloves (finely chopped)
1 head (2 cups) broccoli (chopped)
4 cups cooked spiral pasta
2 tbsp. parmesan cheese
1 lemon

Method:

Cook pasta as per package directions. In large non-stick skillet, sauté garlic in olive oil. Add broccoli and cook until tender crisp. Add cooked pasta and toss with parmesan cheese (and a squeeze of fresh lemon).

Serves 4
200 calories/serving
7 fat units/serving

LENTIL CASSEROLE

Ingredients:

1 ¾ cup lentils
2 cups water
1 tsp. soy sauce
2 cups onions, chopped
2 cloves garlic, minced
1 bay leaf
Salt and pepper to taste
1 tsp. marjoram
1 tsp. sage
1 tsp. thyme
¼ tsp. cayenne

Method:

Simmer lentils, water and bay leaf for 40 minutes; add more water if necessary. Add remaining ingredients and simmer until tender.

Serves 4
225 calories/serving
1 fat unit/serving

LENTILS WITH RICE LOAF

Ingredients:

2 cups cooked lentils
1 cup low-fat bread cubes
½ cup celery, chopped
½ cup onion, chopped
3 tbsp. soy sauce
1 cup long-grain brown rice, cooked
1 tsp. sage
1 tsp. thyme
1 tsp. curry powder
½ cup chicken broth
Pam vegetable spray

Method:

Combine all ingredients. Bake in loaf pan which has been sprayed with Pam. Bake at 350°F for 45 minutes.

Serves 4
180 calories/serving
1 fat unit/serving

LINGUINI WITH ASPARAGUS AND RED PEPPER

Ingredients:

5 cups cooked linguini (10 oz dry)
4 cups asparagus, cut into 4" pieces
1 cup red pepper, coarsely chopped
3 cloves garlic, minced
½ cup fresh parsley, chopped
1 tsp. dried basil
Salt and pepper to taste
1 tbsp. olive oil
½ cup chicken broth

Method:

Cook linguini as directed. Steam red pepper and asparagus in chicken broth. Set aside. Sauté garlic until tender in hot oil; combine with chicken broth mixture. Combine linguini, vegetables, chicken broth mixture and herbs. Serve immediately.

Serves 5
375 calories/serving
1 fat unit/serving

Vegetable chili

Ingredients:

2 cups zucchini, finely chopped
1 cup carrot, finely chopped
1 cup onion, finely chopped
3 cans (14½ oz each) tomatoes, drained and chopped
3 cans (15 oz each) kidney beans
3 cloves garlic, minced
1 tbsp. olive oil
2 tbsp. chili powder
½ tsp. basil
½ tsp. oregano
1/4 tsp. cumin

Method:

Drain and rinse 2 cans kidney beans, set aside. Sauté onion and garlic in hot oil until soft; add spices and mix. Add tomatoes, drained kidney beans and 1 can undrained kidney beans. Bring to a boil; reduce heat and simmer uncovered for 35 minutes or until thickened.

Serves 8 (1 cup servings)
125 calories/serving
3 fat units/serving

VEGETABLE LASAGNA (DELICIOUS!)

Ingredients:

3 cups grated carrots
3 cups grated zucchini
1 cup 1% cottage cheese
3 egg whites, slightly beaten
2 (10 oz) pkg. frozen chopped spinach, thawed and drained
2½ cups spaghetti sauce
½ lb. Lasagna noodles, cooked as per package directions
½ cup skim milk cheese, grated
Pam vegetable spray

Method:

Sauté carrots and zucchini separately in Teflon pan sprayed with Pam. Divide egg whites into 4 even parts; mix 1/4 of the egg white with each of the following: carrots, zucchini, spinach and cottage cheese. Spoon ⅔ cup sauce into medium sized baking pan; place half of the noodles over sauce; top with spinach mixture, then cottage cheese, followed by carrot mixture, then ⅔ cup sauce, followed by zucchini mixture. Top with remaining noodles and sauce. Cover pan and bake at 350°F for 30 minutes. Remove cover and sprinkle with grated cheese; bake 10 minutes longer. Cool 10 minutes before serving.

Serves 6 (large servings)
240 calories/serving
9 fat units/serving

Veggie spaghetti (delicious!)

Ingredients:

1 (700ml) jar "Healthy Choice" or "Too Good To Be True" (President's Choice) pasta sauce
½ cup onions, coarsely chopped
½ cup green pepper, coarsely chopped
½ cup red pepper, coarsely chopped
½ cup fresh green beans, cooked and cut into 2" pieces
1 cup mushrooms, sliced
3 cloves garlic, finely chopped
1 tbsp. vegetable oil
4 tsp. Low-calorie sweetener
Salt and pepper to taste

Method:

Gently simmer pasta sauce. Sauté onions, green and red peppers and garlic in ½ tbsp. hot oil until vegetables are tender; add to pasta sauce. Sauté mushrooms in ½ tbsp. hot oil until lightly browned; add to pasta sauce. Add beans, sweetener and salt and pepper. Simmer for an additional 10 minutes. Serve with spaghetti noodles.

Meat option: add 2oz of browned extra lean ground beef per serving to sautéed mixture. Increases calories to 230 and fat units to 14 per serving. Remember to add the calories and fat units for the pasta you choose (160 calories and 1 fat unit per cup of cooked spaghetti)

Serves 5
80 calories/serving
4 fat units/serving

8. VEGETABLES

RATATOUILLE (DELICIOUS!)

Ingredients:

1 large eggplant, unpeeled and sliced
2 cups leeks, sliced
1 ½ cups red pepper, coarsely chopped
1 ½ cups green pepper, coarsely chopped
3 cups zucchini, sliced
3 cloves garlic, finely chopped
2 cups tomatoes, sliced
1/4 cup fresh parsley, chopped
1 (14 oz) can tomato paste
1 pkg. Chicken broth
1 tsp. Rosemary
1 tsp. Thyme
Salt and pepper to taste
2 tsp. low calorie sweetener

Method:

Place eggplant in a large bowl and add a dash of salt. Add remaining vegetables. Combine broth, sweetener, tomato paste and herbs; mix well. Pour over vegetable mixture; cover and bake at 350°F for 40 minutes.

Serves 8
75 calories/serving
1 fat unit/serving

SWEET 'N SOUR ONIONS

Ingredients:

6–8 medium onions, thickly sliced
1/4 cup boiling water
1/4 tsp. Paprika
1 tsp. Salt
1/4 cup cider vinegar
1/4 cup low calorie sweetener

Method:

Spray casserole dish with Pam spray. Place onions in dish, sprinkle with salt and paprika. Combine vinegar, sweetener and water. Pour over onions and bake uncovered at 350°F for 30 minutes.

Serves 4
12 calories/serving
0 fat units/serving

SUPER SQUASH

Ingredients:

2 large butternut squash
4 tbsp. granulated brown low calorie sweetener (twin)
Salt and pepper to taste
½ tsp. nutmeg

Method:

Pierce squash skin then cook in oven or microwave until well done. Scoop the squash pulp from the outer shell. Mash pulp until smooth and add sweetener and spices to taste. Serve hot.

Serves 6
80 calories/serving
0 fat units/serving

9. POTATOES

DILLED POTATO SALAD

Ingredients:

1½ lbs. potatoes, cooked and quartered (or 3 large potatoes)
⅓ cup green onions, sliced
1½ tsp. dried dill weed
salt and pepper to taste
½ cup no-fat Italian dressing

Method:
Combine dressing, dill and salt and pepper; pour over cooled potatoes and onion. Cover and refrigerate.

Serves 4
160 calories/serving
0 fat units/serving

FRESH BASIL POTATO SALAD

Ingredients:

3 large potatoes, cooked
1 cup no-fat yogurt
2 tbsp. fresh parsley, chopped
1 tbsp. fresh basil chopped or 1 tsp. Dried
1 tbsp. sliced green onion
½ cup frozen peas, thawed
½ cup red pepper, chopped
Salt and pepper to taste

Method:
Cool potatoes and cut into cubes; set aside. Combine yogurt, onion and season with herbs. Add potatoes, peas and red pepper; toss gently until mixed. Cover and refrigerate.

Serves 4
170 calories/serving
0 fat units/serving

NEW POTATOES WITH CUCUMBER DRESSING

Ingredients:

6 medium sized new potatoes, quartered
½ large English cucumber, diced
6 sprigs fresh mint
1 cup no-fat yogurt
Salt and pepper to taste

Method:

Cook potatoes in cold salted water with 2 sprigs of mint. Finely chop remaining mint leaves and add to yogurt. Season yogurt with salt and pepper. Serve hot or cold. If serving cold, chill potatoes 1–2 hours. Add yogurt mixture to potatoes and cucumber just prior to serving. Garnish with mint sprigs.

Serves 6
145 calories/serving
1 fat unit/serving

OLD-FASHIONED POTATO SALAD

Ingredients:

2 cups cubed, cooked potatoes
2 hard-cooked egg whites, chopped
1½ cups celery, chopped
½ cup green onions, chopped
1/4 cup radishes, thinly sliced
1/4 cup sweet pickles, chopped
1½ cups no-fat mayonnaise
3 tbsp. sweet pickle juice
1 tbsp. dijon mustard
Sprinkle of paprika
Salt and pepper to taste

Method:

Combine potatoes, egg whites, celery, onions, radishes and pickles. Set aside. Combine mayonnaise, pickle juice, mustard and salt and pepper. Pour over potato mixture and toss gently until mixed. Garnish with paprika. Cover and refrigerate.

Serves 12
190 calories/serving
1 fat unit/serving

POTATO BOATS

Ingredients:

1 medium sized baked potato
1½ tbsp. no-fat yogurt
2 tsp. onion, finely chopped
1 tsp. dried dill weed or
1 tsp. chives, finely chopped
Sprinkle of garlic powder
Salt and pepper to taste

Method:

Cut potato in half lengthwise; scoop out pulp, leaving skin in tact. Mash pulp; add yogurt, onion and season with herbs. Place combined pulp mixture back into skins. Brown in 400°F oven for 5 minutes.

Makes 2 potato boats
160 calories/2 boats
1 fat unit/2 boats

POTATOES WITH YOGURT

Ingredients:

3 or 4 small new potatoes per serving
2 tbsp. no-fat yogurt per serving
1/8 cup chives, finely chopped
Salt and pepper to taste
Sprinkle of garlic
1 tbsp. fresh parsley, chopped

Method:

Steam or boil potatoes with skins left on. If serving cold, refrigerate for 1–2 hours. Combine yogurt and herbs. Prior to serving, pour yogurt mixture over potatoes. Garnish with additional chives.

168 calories/serving
1 fat unit/serving

YUMMY MASHED POTATOES

Ingredients:

1 large potato per person (8 oz), peeled and cooked
1/4 cup no-fat yogurt per serving
1 tbsp. fresh parsley, chopped
1 tsp. dried dill weed <u>or</u>
1 tsp. chopped chives
Salt and pepper to taste
Sprinkle of garlic powder

Method:

   Mash potato until smooth; add yogurt and season with herbs. Serve immediately.

200 calories/serving (1 cup)
1 fat unit/serving

10. Rice

Curried rice

Ingredients:

1½ cups long-grain brown rice (makes 4 cups cooked rice)
1/4 cup onion, finely chopped
2 cloves garlic, minced
1 stalk celery, finely chopped
2 pkgs. chicken broth (no water added)
1 tsp. rosemary
1 tsp. curry powder
Salt and pepper to taste

Method:

Combine all ingredients with 3 cups water; bring to a boil; reduce heat and simmer over low heat until rice is soft.

Serves 4
170 calories/serving
1 fat unit/serving

Rice pudding (just like mom's)

Ingredients:

1½ cups uncooked long-grain rice
2 cups skim milk
2 egg whites, slightly beaten
2 tsp. granulated brown low calorie sweetener
1/4 cup raisins
1 tsp. cinnamon
1 cup fresh blueberries
1 cup water

Method:

Combine rice, milk and water; cook until rice softens; add remaining ingredients and stir lightly. Can be served warm or cold; if cold, refrigerate 1–2 hours.

Serves 8
135 calories/serving
0 fat units/serving

VEGETABLE RICE

Ingredients:

1½ cups long-grain brown rice (makes 4½ cups cooked)
3 cups water
2 pkgs. chicken broth (no water added)
1/4 cup onion, finely chopped
2 cloves garlic, minced
1/4 cup green pepper, finely chopped
Salt and pepper to taste

Method:

Combine all ingredients; bring to a boil; reduce heat and simmer over low heat until rice is tender.

Serves 4
170 calories/serving
1 fat unit/serving

11. DESSERTS

21 DESSERTS—150 CALORIES AND 3 FAT UNITS (OR LESS)

DESSERT	CALORIES	FAT UNITS
1/2 cup cantaloupe pieces with 3.5 oz frozen yogurt (chocolate, black cherry)	140	3
Delicious frozen yogurt (4 oz) many flavours	125	3
Sugar-free Jello (1 pkg) with sliced banana per 1 cup serving	45	0
No fat yogurt (1 cup) with 1/2 cup fresh raspberries, strawberries and/or blueberries	150	0
2 fresh peaches cut up with skim milk (4 oz) and sprinkled with 1 tsp. low calorie sweetener	120	0
Fresh pineapple pieces - 1 cup	80	1
A big piece of watermelon	60	1
Sugar free Jello whipped with no fat yogurt (total 1 cup) (1/2 and 1/2) topped with 1/4 cup fruit	85	0
1 honey whole wheat raisin bun with 1 Tbsp. Lite jam	145	1
Fresh fruit cocktail - 1 cup	80	0
1 cup green or red seedless grapes	110	1
A large crisp apple cut up in pieces and sprinkled with cinnamon	100	1
1/2 cup 1% cottage cheese with 1/2 cup fruit	120	2
3.5 oz frozen yogurt topped with 1/2 Tbsp. maple syrup	135	3
Frozen Yogurt Float - 10 oz diet drink, 3.5 oz frozen yogurt try - Chocolate & Diet Coke - Blackcherry & Diet Sprite use your imagination!	115	3
4 oz frozen lime, lemon or orange Sherbet with 1/2 Tbsp. Creme de Menthe or Kahlua liqueur	140	2
4 oz 1% Ice Cream - many delicious flavours	120	1
* NO FAT Fruit Flavoured Yogurt (1 cup)	110	0

* New!

APPLE "KELLY"

Ingredients:

1 large apple, peeled and cored
2 tbsp. granulated brown low calorie sweetener
½ tsp. cinnamon

Method:

Combine sweetener and cinnamon; sprinkle over apple and microwave on high power for 3–4 minutes or cook in oven until tender. Serve hot with 2 oz 1% parlor caramel ripple ice cream.

Serves 1
145 calories/serving
.5 fat units/serving

AMY'S CINNAMON APPLESAUCE (DESSERT OR CONDIMENT)

Ingredients:

6 apples, peeled and quartered
1/4 cup water
1 tbsp. lemon juice
3 tbsp. granulated brown low calorie sweetener
1 tsp. cinnamon

Method:

In saucepan, combine apples, water and lemon juice. Bring to a boil, reduce heat and simmer gently uncovered until apples are tender (about 15 minutes). Stir often. Mash or process until puree. Add sweetener and cinnamon. Mix well.

Serves 6
100 calories/serving
.5 fat units/serving

PEARS IN RED WINE

Ingredients:

6 ripe pears, peeled and left whole
½ tsp. cinnamon or ground ginger
4 tbsp. granulated brown low calorie sweetener
1 cup red wine
1/4 cup water

Method:

Combine all ingredients (except pears) and bring to a boil in saucepan. Place pears in a deep dish, pour wine sauce on top and cover with saran wrap. Microwave on high for about 5 minutes or just tender. Or place pears in a saucepan with wine sauce and simmer for 10–15 minutes, turning pears carefully to ensure even coloring. Serve hot or cold.

Serves 6
120 calories/serving
1 fat unit/serving

Chapter 17

Food Lists—Index

Index

1.	Drinks/beverages	162
2.	Dairy products/eggs	162/163
3.	Grain foods–bread, cereals, crackers, flour	163
4.	Meat (beef, lamb, pork, etc.)	164
5.	Poultry (chicken, turkey, duck)	164
6.	Seafood/fish	164
7.	Pasta/rice/beans	165
8.	Vegetables	165
9.	Fruits/juices	165/166
10.	Cooking oils/fats/spreads	166
11.	Salad dressings	166
12.	Nuts/seeds	167
13.	Fast foods/sweets/desserts	167/168
14.	Miscellaneous condiments/pickles/sauces/soups	168

For a great pocket reference we suggest you purchase the American Heart Association's "Fat and Cholesterol Counter" available at book stores for less than $5.00.

* Reference for food lists: Pennington, J.: Bowes & Church's Food Values of Portions commonly used, 1989, J.B. Lippincott Co., New York.

1 Fat Unit = 1 Gram of Fat = 9 Calories

	AMT	CAL	FAT UNITS		AMT	CAL	FAT UNITS
1. **DRINKS/BEVERAGES**				**2.** **DAIRY PRODUCTS**			
Water	8 oz	0	0	Butter	1 tbsp	100	11
Milk				*Cheese*			
3.5%	8 oz	150	8	Cheddar	1 oz	115	9
2%	8 oz	120	4.5	Colby	1 oz	110	9
1%	8 oz	100	2.5	Cottage Cheese- (regular)	½ cup	120	5
Skim	8 oz	85	0	Cottage Cheese- (1%)	½ cup	80	1
Buttermilk	8 oz	100	2	Creamed Cheese	1 tbsp	50	5
				Creamed Cheese- (light)	1 tbsp	32	2.5
Regular soft drinks (sodas)	12 oz	155	0	Edam	1 oz	100	8
Diet soft drinks	12 oz	1	0	Feta	1 oz	75	6
				Mozzarella (reg.)	1 oz	80	6
tea	6 oz	2	0	Swiss	1 oz	105	8
coffee · instant/brewed	6 oz	2	0	*Light Cheeses	1 oz	50	2
				Cheese spreads	1 oz	70	5
Fruit Juices							
apple	8 oz	130	0	*Cream*			
orange	8 oz	130	0	Table Cream	1 oz	60	6
lemonade	8 oz	130	0	Half & Half	1 oz	40	3
Alcoholic Beverages				Sour Cream(light)	1 tbsp	26	2.5
Beer	12 oz	150	0	1% Sour Cream	1 tbsp	13	.2
Light Beer	12 oz	100	0				
80 proof (rum, vodka, gin, whisky)	1½oz	100	0	Whipped Cream Whipped	1 cup	800	88
wine (red, white, rose)	4 oz	80	0	Cream- (light)	1 cup	700	74
				Imitation Whipped Cream (Cool Whip)	1 cup	200	16
				Eggs			
				1 large	1	80	6
				1 white	1	16	0
				1 yolk	1	63	6
				Egg Beaters	2 oz	25	0
				Frozen Dairy Products			
				Frozen Yogurt(reg)	4 oz	140	3
				Frozen Yogurt(no-fat)	4 oz	100	0

	AMT	CAL	FAT UNITS		AMT	CAL	FAT UNITS
Frozen Dairy Products - cont'd.				**Bread Rolls**			
				Hot Dog/ Hamburger	1	110	2
Ice Cream				Dinner Rolls (2½")	1	90	2
Rich Chocolate	4 oz	250	17				
Regular Strawberry	4 oz	130	6	_Cereals_			
1% Butterscotch	4 oz	110	1	(add milk calories/fat			
				units)			
Milk							
See Beverages - pg. 162				Bran Crunchies	¾cup	115	1
				Bran Flakes	¾cup	115	1
Milkshake				Corn Bran	⅔cup	110	1
Thick Strawberry	10 oz	350	8	Corn Grits(Hominy)	1cup	140	1
				100% Natural Granola	1cup	140	.5
Yogurt				Oatmeal	⅔cup	110	2
Regular (fruit)	6 oz	200	6				
Low Fat (fruit)	6 oz	180	2	_Crackers_			
No-Fat plain	6 oz	80	0	Cheese & Peanut Butter	6	200	11
No-Fat (fruit)	6 oz	80	0	Graham (4 sections)	1	60	2
				Ritz	6	100	6
				Saltine	6	72	1
3.				Cracked Wheat	4	60	2
GRAIN FOODS -				Wasa Crisps	2	80	0
BREAD, CEREALS,							
CRACKERS, FLOUR				_Flour_			
				Corn Meal	1cup	500	2
Breads				Rye	1cup	420	3
				White Pastry	1cup	430	1
Bagel (5")	1	160	2	White Enriched	1cup	500	1.5
				Whole Wheat	1cup	400	2.5
English Muffin	1	140	1				
Bread							
French (1" slice)	1	100	1				
Raisin (1/2" slice)	1	70	1				
Rye (1/2" slice)	1	70	1				
Whole Wheat (1/2" slice)	1	70	1				
White (1/2" slice)	1	70	1				
Muffins							
Medium (Donut Shop)	1	260	14				
Low Fat Muffins - pg.97-99	1	120	2				
Croissant (medium)	1	240	12				

	AMT	CAL	FAT UNITS		AMT	CAL	FAT UNITS
4.				_Turkey_			
MEATS (beef, lamb, pork,				light meat w/o skin	1 oz	40	1.5
etc. roasted)				dark meat w/o skin	1 oz	54	2
				light & dark w/skin	1 oz	60	4
Ground Beef							
extra lean (Can.)	1 oz	55	3	_Duck_			
extra lean (U.S.)	1 oz	65	5	without skin	1 oz	60	3
lean	1 oz	75	6	with skin	1 oz	90	8
regular	1 oz	90	8				
Sirloin Steak ·				**6.**			
broiled-lean only	1 oz	70	4	**FISH/SEAFOOD**			
lean & fat	1 oz	80	5				
				Fish			
T-Bone	1 oz	90	7	Bass	1 oz	30	1
				Cod	1 oz	30	.5
Beef Sausage	1 oz	90	8	Grouper	1 oz	25	.5
				Haddock	1 oz	25	.5
Lamb				Herring (pickled)	1 pce	65	4
Leg of Lamb ·				Mackerel	1 oz	60	.4
lean & fat	1 oz	75	5	Perch	1 oz	25	.5
lean only	1 oz	55	3	Salmon	1 oz	50	3
lean Lamb Chop	1 oz	70	4	Snapper	1 oz	30	.5
				Sole	1 oz	25	.5
Pork				Trout	1 oz	30	1
Bacon	1 slc.	40	3	Tuna	1 oz	40	1.5
Ham ·				Tuna in oil	1 oz	65	4
lean & fat	1 oz	80	6	Tuna in water	1 oz	30	1
lean only	1 oz	60	3	Whitefish	1 oz	40	2
Loin ·							
lean & fat	1 oz	90	7	_Seafood_			
lean only	1 oz	70	4	Clams	1 oz	40	1
					½ cup	120	2
Pork Sausage	1 oz	110	10	Crab	1 oz	25	.5
				Lobster	1 oz	25	.5
Beaver (we are healthy	1 oz	50	2	Mussels	1 oz	25	1
Canucks!)					½ cup	65	3
				Octopus	1 oz	20	.5
				Oysters	1 oz	40	1.5
5.					½ cup	90	3
POULTRY (roasted)				Scallops (2 lrg)	1 oz	25	.5
				Shrimp	1 oz	30	.5
Chicken					4 lge	30	.5
light meat w/o skin	1 oz	50	1.5				
dark meat w/o skin	1 oz	60	3				
light & dark w/skin	1 oz	70	4				

	AMT	CAL	FAT UNITS		AMT	CAL	FAT UNITS
7. PASTA/RICE/BEANS				Vegetables-cont'd.			
				Onions - raw	1cup	50	0
Pasta				Parsnips	1cup	100	0
Macaroni	1cup	160	1	Peas - cooked	1cup	130	0
Egg Noodles	1cup	200	2	Peppers (green or red)	1cup	25	0
Macaroni & Cheese (prepackaged)	1cup	380	17	Potatoes (baked or broiled) 1 medium with skin	5 oz	100	0
Linguini	1cup	200	2	1 medium no skin	5 oz	90	0
Spaghetti	1cup	160	1	Pumpkin	1cup	50	0
				Radishes	½cup	10	0
Rice				Sauerkraut	1cup	45	0
Brown	1cup	200	0	Soybeans	1cup	300	11
White (parboiled)	1cup	200	0	Tofu (3"x3"x1")	1 pce	125	8
Wild Rice	1cup	180	0	Spinach - cooked	1cup	40	0
				Squash - cooked			
Beans				Zucchini	1cup	40	0
Baked Beans (canned)	1cup	250	4	Acorn, Butternut	1cup	80	0
Kidney Beans	1cup	225	1	Sweet Potatoes - cooked with skin	1cup	340	0
Lima Beans	1cup	220	1	Tomatoes -			
Navy Beans	1cup	260	1	1 medium raw	1	25	0
Yellow Beans	1cup	250	2	1 cup pieces	1cup	35	0
Lentils	1cup	230	1	Tomato Juice	1cup	45	0
Chick Peas	1cup	270	2	Tomato Sauce	1cup	75	0
Blackeyed Peas	1cup	200	1	Turnips	1cup	30	0
8. VEGETABLES				**9. FRUITS/JUICES**			
Asparagus	1cup	40	0				
Beets	1cup	50	0	Apple - 1 medium	1	80	0
Broccoli	1cup	50	0	Apple juice	8 oz	120	0
Cabbage	1cup	30	0	Applesauce - (unsweetened)	4 oz	50	0
Carrots - raw	1cup	50	0	Apricots - 3 medium	3	50	0
Carrots - cooked	1cup	70	0	Apricots - fresh	1cup	70	0
Cauliflower	1cup	25	0	Banana	1med	105	0
Chard - cooked	1cup	35	0	Blackberries	1cup	75	0
Corn	1 ear	80	1	Blueberries	1cup	80	0
Corn - cream style	1cup	180	1	Cantaloupe	1cup	55	0
Corn - kernels	1cup	180	2	Cantaloupe ½ medium	½	90	0
Cucumber	1cup	15	0	Cherries - sour pitted	1cup	80	0
Garlic	1 clv.	5	0	Cherries - sweet fresh	12	60	1
Lettuce - raw	1cup	5	0				
Mushrooms	1cup	20	0				

	AMT	CAL	FAT UNITS		AMT	CAL	FAT UNITS
Fruit/Juices · cont'd.				Cooking Oils · Cont'd.			
Cranberry · juice	8 oz	145	0	Margarine	½ cup	815	90
Cranberry · sauce	½ cup	210	0		1 tbsp	102	11.5
Fruit Cocktail ·					1 tsp	34	4
canned in water	1 cup	80	0				
heavy syrup	1 cup	180	0	Diet Margarine	½ cup	408	48
1/2 grapefruit	1/2	40	0		1 tbsp	50	5.5
Grapes ·					1 tsp	17	2
seedless green	1 cup	60	0				
juice	8 oz	150	0	Peanut Butter	1 tbsp	95	8
Lemon · medium	1	20	0				
Nectarine	1	70	0	*Animal Fats/Oils*			
Orange	1	60	0	Butter	½ cup	864	96
Orange Juice	8 oz	120	0		1 tbsp	108	12
Peaches ·	1 med	40	0		1 tsp	36	4
canned in water	1 cup	60	0				
canned in syrup	1 cup	190	0	Light Butter	1 tbsp	54	6
Pears ·	1 med	90	0		1 tsp	18	2
canned in water	1 cup	70	0				
canned in syrup	1 cup	180	0	Lard (Pork)	½ cup	928	104
Pineapple · fresh	1 cup	70	0		1 tbsp	116	13
canned in water	1 cup	80	0				
canned in syrup	1 cup	190	0				
Plums · fresh	1	40	0	11.			
canned in syrup	1 cup	180	0	**SALAD DRESSINGS**			
Raisins · seedless	1 cup	500	8				
Raspberries	1 cup	60	0	*Mayonnaise*			
Rhubarb · fresh	1 cup	40	0	Regular	½ cup	800	89
Strawberries · fresh	1 cup	45	0		1 tbsp	100	11
Tangerine · fresh	1	30	0	Light	1 tbsp	50	5.5
Watermelon	1 cup	48	0	No-Fat	1 tbsp	12	0
10.				*Salad Dressing*			
COOKING OILS /				Regular ·			
FATS / SPREADS				Blue Cheese	1 tbsp	80	8
				Caesar	1 tbsp	80	6
Vegetable Oils				French	1 tbsp	67	6.5
All vegetable oils	1 tbsp	120	13	Italian	1 tbsp	70	7
(Sunflower, Safflower,	½ cup	960	105	Thousand Island	1 tbsp	60	5.5
Olive, Peanut, Canola	(4oz)						
				Low Calorie·			
Shortening	½ cup	848	96	French	1 tbsp	22	1
	1 tsp	106	12	Italian	1 tbsp	16	1.5
				Thousand Island	1 tbsp	24	1.5

	AMT	CAL	FAT UNITS		AMT	CAL	FAT UNITS
Salad Dressing -cont'd.				**13.**			
				FAST FOODS /			
No Fat ·				**SNACKS / SWEETS**			
French	1 tbsp	15	0				
Italian	1 tbsp	5	0	Apple Pie	1	300	14
Thousand Island	1 tbsp	30	0	Baked Potato · plain	1	200	0
				Baked Potato · bacon & cheese	1	400	12
12.				Bacon Double Cheeseburger	1	500	31
NUTS AND SEEDS				Brownie	1	250	11
				Cake · small w/icing	2 oz	200	12
Nuts				Cheeseburger · single	1	320	15
Almonds · slivered	½ cup	400	35	Chicken Burger	1	470	20
Almonds · 20 nuts	1 oz	150	15	Chicken Dinner ·	1	700	43
				(2 pc. deep fried)			
Cashews · Roasted	½ cup	400	31	Chicken Nuggets	6	275	17
Cashews · 20 nuts	1 oz	170	14	Chicken salad with croissant	1	460	36
Coconut · shredded	½ cup	150	14	English Muffin with egg and cheese	1	340	16
Mixed Nuts	½ cup	400	32	English Muffin with cheese and sausage	1	500	32
	1 oz	170	14	Fries (regular)	1	230	12
Peanuts · 30 nuts	1 oz	150	14	Hamburger Deluxe · (2 patties)	1	520	30
Peanuts	½ cup	400	32	Onion Rings (reg.)	1	280	16
Pecans · 12 halves	1 oz	190	19	Pancake Platter with syrup and butter	1	440	15
Seeds				Pizza (pep & cheese)	2 slc.	450	14
Poppy	1 tbsp	45	3	Roast Beef Sandwich	1	310	12
				Sundae w/fudge and peanuts	1	700	40
Sunflower · shelled	1 oz	160	14	Shake (10 oz choc.)	1	360	11
	1 tbsp	45	4	Scrambled egg Platter	1	460	30
				*Turkey Sub no mayo or butter (small bun)	1	300	6
				Candy/Chocolate			
				Chocolate Bar · (1.5 · 2 oz)	1	300	20
				Bridge Mixture · (14)	1 oz	140	6
				Chocolate Almonds · (8 pieces)	1 oz	160	12
				Life Savers	1	10	0
				Mints	¼ cup	100	1

	AMT	CAL	FAT UNITS		AMT	CAL	FAT UNITS
Fast Foods / Snacks / Sweets · Cont'd.				*Commercial Soups*			
				Broth Based	8 oz	70	2
Cookies				Chunky	8 oz	150	5
Chocolate Chip · 3	1 oz	150	8	Creamed	8 oz	120	7.5
Ginger Snaps · 5	1 oz	100	3	Clam Chowder	8 oz	90	2
Granola Bar · Peanut Butter w/choc. chips	1 oz	130	5	Noodle	8 oz	70	2
				Wonton	8 oz	40	1
Oatmeal Raisin · 2	1 oz	140	6				
Peanut Butter · 2	1 oz	150	8				
Sugar · 2	1 oz	140	6				
Ice Cream Treats							
Rich Choc. Ice cream Bar	1	360	25				
Frozen Yogurt Bar	1	90	3				
Pies							
Apple/Cherry-med. pc.	1	400	17				
Pecan · med. pc.	1	600	32				
Others							
Chocolate Mousse	1 cup	600	40				
Sugar Donut · med.	1	275	14				
Commercial Muffin · medium	1	260	14				
14. MISCELLANEOUS							
Beef or Chicken Broth	1 cup	25	0				
Broth Cube	cube	6	0				
Cornstarch	1 tbsp	30	0				
Ketchup	1 tbsp	15	0				
Mustard	1 med	15	0				
Pickles · dill	1	6	0				
Pickles · sweet	1 tsp	18	0				
Pepper	1 tsp	5	0				
Salt	¼ cup	0	0				
Soya Sauce	1 tbsp	24	0				
	1 tbsp	6	0				
Worcestershire Sauce	1 tbsp	10	0				
Vinegar	1	1	0				

CHAPTER 18

WRAP-UP

Congratulations readers! We are on our way to health *and* vitality with lean, fit bodies! Every reader can succeed on *"The Final Diet."* We are knowledgeable and prepared.

A REVIEW:

1. Fat has 9 calories/gram compared to 4 calories/gram for protein and carbohydrate.
2. A human body that is fed a low fat diet metabolizes body fat and gets thinner!
3. The human body needs:
   Over 60% of calories as carbohydrates
   15% of calories (approximately 70 grams) as protein
   15–20% (or less) of calories as fat
4. Complex carbohydrates are wonderful–the body's favorite fuel nutritious, filling and healthy.
5. We must eat three or more filling meals a day–but we must eat the right food.
6. We must make smart substitutions!
7. We must exercise—45 minutes–four times a week.

AND FINALLY:

- When you reach your ideal weight, make "The Final Diet" you "life Diet"
- Exercise…for life!

BIBLIOGRAPHY

AMERICAN HEART ASSOCIATION: FAT & CHOLESTEROL COUNTER, RANDOM HOUSE, NEW YORK, 1991.

ANDREWS, J. F.: "EXERCISE FOR SLIMMING." PROCEEDINGS OF THE NUTRITION SOCIETY (1991), 50.

BARNETT, ROB'T.: "WHY FAT MAKES YOU FATTER." AMERICAN HEALTH, MAY 1986.

BELLERSON, KAREN J.: "THE FAT BOOK." AVERY PUBLISHING, GROUP NEW YORK, 1991.

BRAY, GEORGE A.: "TREATMENT FOR OBESITY: A NUTRIENT BALANCE/NUTRIENT PARTITION APPROACH." NUTRITIONAL REVIEWS, FEB. 1991, VOL. 49, #2.

BRODY, JANE: "GOOD FOOD BOOK—LIVING THE HIGH CARBOHYDRATE WAY." 1987, W. W. NORTON, NEW YORK.

BROWNELL, KELLY D.: "BEHAVIOR MODIFICATION AND RELAPSE PREVENTION." CONTEMPORARY MANAGEMENT OF THE OVERWEIGHT PATIENT, UNIVERSITY OF WASHINGTON SCHOOL OF MEDICINE, NUMBER 4, SUMMER 92.

CASTELLI, W. P. ET AL.: "INCIDENCE OF CORONARY HEART DISEASE AND CHOLESTEROL LEVELS—THE FRAMING HAM STUDY." JOURNAL OF THE AMERICAN MEDICAL ASSOCIATION, VOL. 256, 1986.

CILISKA, D.: "WOMEN AND OBESITY, LEARNING TO LIVE WITH IT." CAN. FAMILY PHYSICIAN JOURNAL, JAN. 1993, VOL. 39.

CRAIGHEAD, L. W.: "MECHANISMS OF ACTION IN COGNITIVE—BEHAVIORAL AND PHARMACOLOGICAL INTERVENTIONS FOR OBESITY AND BULIMIA." JOURNAL OF CONSULTING AND CLINICAL PSYCHOLOGY. 1991. VOL. 59, #1.

COOPER, KENNETH: "THE NEW AEROBICS." 1983, BANTAM BOOKS, NEW YORK.

COOPER, KENNETH ET AL.: "THE NEW AEROBICS FOR WOMEN." 1988, BANTAM BOOKS, NEW YORK.

DOUGHERTY, R. M. ET AL.: "NUTRIENT CONTENT OF THE DIET WHEN THE FAT IS REDUCED." AMERICAN JOURNAL OF CLINICAL NUTRITION, 1988. VOLUME 48.

FOREGT, JOHN P.: "FACTORS COMMON TO SUCCESSFUL THERAPY FOR THE OBESE PATIENT." MEDICINE AND SCIENCE IN SPORTS AND MEDICINE, 1991, VOL. 23, #3.

FRICKER, J. ET AL.: "ENERGY—METABOLISM ADAPTATION IN OBESE ADULTS ON A VERY LOW CALORIE DIET." AMERICAN JOURNAL OF CLINICAL NUTRITION, APRIL 1991, VOL. 53, #4.

GARBER, A. M. ET AL.: "SCREENING ASYMPTOMATIC ADULTS FOR CARDIAC RISK FACTORS: THE SERUM CHOLESTEROL LEVEL." ANNALS INTERNAL MEDICINE. 1989. VOL. 110, #8.

GODRICK, G. K. ET AL.: "WHY TREATMENTS FOR OBESITY DON'T LAST." JOURNAL OF THE AMERICAN DIETETICS ASSOC., OCT. 1991, VOL. 9, #10.

GOLD, PHIL ET AL.: "CHOLESTEROL AND CORONARY HEART DISEASE—THE GREAT DEBATE" 1992, PANTHENON PUBLISHING GROUP LTD., PARK RIDGE, NEW JERSEY.

GOOR, RON ET AL.: "THE CHOOSE TO LOSE DIET." 1990, HOUGHTON MIFFLIN CO., BOSTON, MASSACHUSETTS.

GREENSPAN, F. S.: "BASIC & CLINICAL ENDOCRINOLOGY, 3RD EDITION." 1991, APPLETON-LANGE, NORWALK, CONNECTICUT.

GRUNDY, SCOTT M. ET AL.: "AMERICAN HEART ASSOCIATIONS, LOW-FAT, LOW-CHOLESTEROL COOKBOOK." 1989. RANDOM HOUSE INC. NEW YORK.

HAMMER, R. L. ET AL.: "CALORIE RESTRICTED LOW-FAT DIET AND EXERCISE IN OBESE WOMEN." AMERICAN JOURNAL OF CLINICAL NUTRITION 49, 1989.

HEALTH AND WELFARE CANADA: "NUTRITION RECOMMENDATIONS, THE REPORT OF THE SCIENTIFIC REVIEW COMMITTEE." 1990, CANADIAN GOVERNMENT PUBLISHING, OTTAWA, CANADA.

KATAHN, MARTIN: "THE T-FACTOR DIET." 1990, BANTAM, NEW YORK.

KAVANAGH, T.: "TAKE HEART." 1992, KEY PORTER BOOKS, TORONTO.

KINSELLA, J. B. ET AL.: "DIETARY N-3 POLYUNSATURATED FATTY ACIDS AND THE AMELIORATION OF CARDIOVASCULAR DISEASE." AMERICAN JOURNAL CLINICAL NUTRITION, VOL. 52.

KISSEBACH, A. H. ET AL: "HEALTH RISKS OF OBESITY." MED. CLINICS OF N. AMERICA, 1989, VOL. 73.

LAPPE, FRANCIS: "DIET FOR A SMALL PLANET." BALLANTINE BOOKS, 1991.

LEITER, L. A.: "DIABETES AND OBESITY." CAN. DIABETES 1988; VOL. 1 (4).

MACDONALD, H. B., HOWARD H.: EAT WELL, LIVE WELL. "THE CANADIAN DIETITIANS GUIDE TO HEALTHY EATING." MACMILLAN OF CANADA, 1990.

MANSON, J. E. ET AL.: "BODY WEIGHT AND LONGEVITY." JOURNAL OF THE AMERICAN MEDICAL ASSOCIATION, 257, 1987.

MCWILLIAMS, JOHN AND PETER: "THE PORTABLE LIFE 101." PRELUDE PRESS, 1992. LOS ANGELES.

MEYERS, MARTIN G.: "CARDIOVASCULAR EFFECTS OF CAFFEINE." CAN FAM PHYSICIAN, JUNE 1992, VOL. 38.

MILES, DANIEL S.: "WEIGHT CONTROL AND EXERCISE." CLINICS IN SPORTS MEDICINE, JAN. 1991, VOLUME 10, #1.

THE MULTIPLE RISK FACTOR INTERVENTION TRIAL RESEARCH GROUP (1990): "MORTALITY RATES AFTER 10-15 YEARS FOR PARTICIPANTS IN THE MULTIPLE RISK FACTOR INTERVENTION TRIAL." JOURNAL AMERICAN MEDICAL ASSOCIATION, 1990, 263.

MURRAY, R. K.: "HARPER'S BIOCHEMISTRY." APPLETON & LANG, 1990.

NICOLIS, R. J. ET AL.: "N-3 FATTY ACIDS AND ATHEROSCLEROSIS." CUNN OPIN. LIPIDOLOGY. 1990, VOL. 1.

PENNINGTON, JEAN A.: "BOWES & CHURCH'S FOOD VALUES OF PORTIONS COMMONLY USED." FIFTEENTH EDITION, 1989, J. B. LIPPINCOTT CO., NEW YORK.

PISCATELLA, JOSEPH C.: "CONTROLLING YOUR FAT TOOTH." 1991. WORKMAN PUBLISHING CO., NEW YORK.

POTENZA, D. P. ET AL.: "ASPARTAME: CLINICAL UPDATE." CONNECTICUT MEDICINE, JULY 1989, VOLUME 53, #7.

RENWICK, A. G.: "ACCEPTABLE DAILY INTAKE OF AND THE REGULATION OF INTENSE SWEETENERS." FOOD ADDITIVES AND CONTAMINANTS. 1990, VOL. 7, #4.

RIPPE, J. M. ET AL.: "WALKING FOR HEALTH AND FITNESS." JOURNAL OF THE AMERICAN MEDICAL ASSOCIATION 259, 1988.

RIPPE, J. M.: "THE EXERCISE EXCHANGE PROGRAM." 1992. SIMON & SHUSTER, NEW YORK.

ROBERTS, W. C (ED.): "THE HYPERTRIGLYCEREMIAS: RISK AND MANAGEMENT." AMERICAN JOURNAL OF CARDIOLOGY. JULY 24, 1991, ENTIRE ISSUE.

ROSSER, W. W.: "ADVISING PATIENTS ABOUT LOW FAT DIETS." CANADIAN FAMILY PHYSICIAN JOURNAL, AN. 1993, VOL. 39.

SHEATS, CLIFFE: "LEAN BODIES." 1992, THE SUMMIT GROUP, FORTH WORTH, TEXAS.

WADDEN, T. A. ET AL: "RESPONSIBLE AND IRRESPONSIBLE USE OF VERY-LOW CALORIE DIETS IN OBESITY." JAN. 1990. VOL. 263.

WILLARD, M. D.: "OBESITY: TYPES AND TREATMENTS." AMERICAN FAMILY PHYSICIAN, JUNE 1991. VOL. 43, #6.

WOOLEY, S. C. ET AL.: "OBESITY TREATMENT: THE HIGH COST OF FALSE HOPE." JOURNAL OF THE AMERICAN DIETETIC ASSOC. OCT. 1991, VOL. 91, #10.

YOST, DAVID A.: "CLINICAL SAFETY OF ASPARTAME." AMERICAN FAMILY PRACTICE, FEB. 1987, VOL. 39, #2.

INDEX

Alcohol drinks 13–18, 162
Aspartame 59–60
Beans 32, 38, 165
Beef 42, 45, 164
Beer 13, 162
Beverages. *See Drinks*
Bread 32–33, 54–60, 163
  spreads 34, 54–60, 166, 168
  whole wheat honey raisin bread 95
Breast feeding 31
Broth 168
Butter 44, 53–60, 162, 166
Buttermilk 162
Calcium
  body's needs 46, 81
Calories, Calorie goal
  tables by body weight 25, 26
Cancer *12*
Candy. *See Sweets*
Carbohydrate
  benefits of 10–18, 32–40
  the body's use of 10–18
  complex carbohydrates 11–18
  initial bloating and 40
  types & complete discussion of 11–18
Cellulose 11
Cereals 11, 35, 163

Cheese
  low fat cheese 47, 162
  1% cottage cheese 46, 48, 62
  regular cheese 47, 162
  skim milk cheese 47, 162
Chicken
  bird of paradise 41–45, 164
Children, The Final Diet and 30–31
Cholesterol
  in food 72
  reduction 72
Coffee 58, 162
Cookies 51, 167
Crackers 163
Cream 58, 162
Dairy products 46–49, 162, 163
  frozen dairy products 47, 162, 163
  ice cream treats 47, 52, 57, 162, 163
  low fat dairy products 46–49
  sour cream 49, 162
Diabetes 20
Diet
  the body's needs 13
  "The Final Diet" 13
  typical north American 13
Donuts *168*
Drinks 58–60, 162, 163
Eggs 73, 162
Exercise 19, 27, 65–71
  aerobic 69–70
  anaerobic 70–71
  benefits of 65
  and calories 66–71
  the second essential 65–71
Family support 19
Fast foods 52–60, 167
Fat unit
  fat unit goals 21–31, 24–28
  grams and 21
  introduction to 21
Fat/hydrogenated 6–7
  the body's use of 4
  monounsaturated 5
  polyunsaturated 5
  saturated 5, 72, 164, 165

traps 50–60
Fiber
  high fiber, benefits of 11, 32–40
The final diet
  game plan 21–31
  principles 74
  questions about 75–77
  weight loss 76–77
Fish
  calories 164
  turkey of the sea 43–44
Flour *34*, 163
Frame size, determining 22
Fruit juices 39, 58, 59, 162, 165, 166
Fruits 39, 165, 166
Goodies. *See Junk food*
Grain products 32–33, 33–35, 163
Heart disease xiii
  cholesterol and 72
High blood pressure xiii
High fat diet, example of 29
High fiber. *See Fiber: high fiber, benefits of*
Ice cream 49, 162, 163
  1% ice cream 49, *162, 163*
Ideal weight, tables by height 25
Juice, fruit 39, 58, 59, 162, 165, 166
Junk food 50, 51, 167, 168
Ketchup 168
Lamb 42, *164*, 165
Lentils 38, 165
Margarine 6, 53–60, 166
Mayonnaise, low fat xiv, 55, 61, 166
Meal plans
  two weeks of great dining 78–83
Milk
  1% milk 46–49, 58, 162
  regular 46–49, 58–60, 162
  skim 46–49, 58, 162
Milkshake 163, 167
Muffins 168
Mustard 168
Nuts 168
Obese
  frequency xiii
  prevention rules 62

Oils, vegetable 5–6, 166
Olive oil 6, 166
Pasta 32, 37
  George's broccoli & garlic 37, 143
Peanut butter 53, 54
Pepper 168
Pickles 168
Pies 61, 167
Pork 42, 164
Potatoes 35–36, 165
  French fries 36
Poultry 41–45, 164
Pregnancy, The Final Diet and 30–31
Protein
  animal 9, 41–45
  the body's use of 7–18
  daily requirement 8, 45
  dairy products and 46–49, 47
  smart substitutions 62
  vegetable 9
Recipe Index 91–94
Recipes. *See Recipe Index*
  appetizers/dips 103
  beef 141, 148
  chicken 131
  desserts 158, 159, 160
  eggs 101, 102
  main courses 124–125
  pork 140
  seafood/fish 136
  soups 106
  turkey 124–125
  20 delicious low fat desserts 158
Restaurants
  survival guide 63–64
Rice 36, 165
Salad dressings 55–60, 61, 166
  no fat 56, 61, 166
Seeds 167
Sherbet 49, 62
The slim six (low fat dairy products 46–49, 62
Snack food 50–60, 61, 167, 168
  great snack food 51, 61, 167, 168
Soft drinks 58, 162

Soups
  commercial 168
  homemade. See Recipes: soups
Soy sauce 168
Spreads 53–60, 61, 166
Starch 11
Stroke xiii
Substitutions
  smart substitutions 61, 62
Sugar 39
Super seven complex carbohydrates 32–40
Sweeteners 59–60
Sweets. *See Junk food*
Tea 58, 162
The slim six 46–49
Thermogenesis 12
Turkey
  bird of paradise 41–45, 164
Vegetables 38, 165
Vinegar 168
Weight, ideal body 21–31
Worcestershire sauce 168
Yogurt
  frozen 46–49, 162, 163
  no-fat 46–49, 162, 163

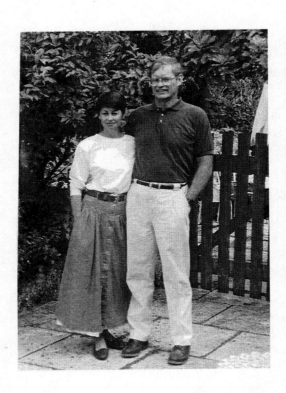

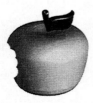 # The Authors

Michael Chatterson is an experienced Family Physician/Emergency Physician who has counselled and treated many thousands of patients with obesity and related problems. He has meticulously researched all of the scientific material in this book. He enjoys reading, writing and teaching. He remains fit and active with basketball, cycling, skiing, Nautilus, and **The Final Diet**.

Linda Schalin Chatterson is a Registered Nurse, mother and homemaker. She has a lifetime interest in nutrition. She created and sampled all off the 100 excellent recipes in the book. She remains fit and active by following **The Final Diet** in combination with cycling, tennis and cross-country skiing.